ACUPUNCTURE

ACUPUNCTURE

What it is, How it Works
and How it Can Help You

RUTH LEVER KIDSON

Sphinx House

Fourth edition, revised and updated, Sphinx House Publishing 2023

First published by Penguin Books Ltd. 1987 under the title *Acupuncture for Everyone*

Second edition (first American edition) by Healing Arts Press 2000

Third edition (second American edition) by Healing Arts Press 2008 under the title *Is Acupuncture Right for You?*

In memory of
Tom Dummer and Marie Ross
who first led me into the world of
complementary medicine

NOTES

ON LANGUAGE

The terms 'he' and 'she' (and 'him' and 'her') are used more or less alternately throughout the book when describing acupuncturists, doctors and patients. This does not imply that either sex is more likely to suffer from a particular condition (unless expressly stated) or to be either acupuncturists or doctors – it is simply to avoid using the ungrammatical 'they' and 'them' to refer to a single individual.

GLOSSARY

For convenience, a few 'medical' words have been used throughout the text. They are:

medial – closest to the midline
lateral – furthest from the midline
distal – furthest from the trunk (eg the foot is the distal part of the leg)
chronic – long standing
acute – occurring suddenly and lasting a short time
humerus – the bone of the upper arm
radius – the bone in the lower arm on the side of the thumb.
ulna – the bone in the lower arm on the side of the little finger

DIAGRAMS AND DESCRIPTIONS OF ACUPUNCTURE POINTS

Please note that this book is not intended to be a do-it-yourself manual, and should not be used as such. The diagrams and descriptions give an approximate guide to the position of the points. The purpose of the book is to be an introduction for people who are receiving treatment, or thinking of receiving treatment, from a qualified acupuncturist, as well as for those who are thinking of training as acupuncturists. For readers who wish to study the therapy in depth, a list of acupuncture colleges is given in the last chapter.

Contents

1

A SHORT HISTORY OF ACUPUNCTURE

Acupuncture has been around for well over two thousand years, and is one of the oldest therapies there is. The theory on which it is based is also the theory that underlies Chinese herbal medicine and although, inevitably, it has developed and changed in certain respects over the centuries, its fundamental principles are still much the same as they were two millennia ago.

THE NEIJING SUWEN

The oldest known book on the theory of Chinese medicine is the *Huangdi Neijing Suwen* (often just referred to as the *Neijing Suwen*). It is still in print today and has been translated into English as *The Yellow Emperor's Classic of Internal Medicine.* Traditionally, the Yellow Emperor of the title was said to have lived in the twenty seventh century BCE – but it seems more likely that he is a semi-mythical character, perhaps one originally based on a real person but, over the centuries, having been endowed with far more greatness than he actually warranted.

However, real person or not, it is highly unlikely that the *Neijing Suwen* in its present form can be attributed to the Yellow Emperor or even dated to his reign. In the twenty seventh century BCE, written Chinese was still in a fairly primitive form known as archaic, or prehistoric, ideographs. But the *Neijing Suwen* is an extremely profound work, and it would have been impossible for it to have been expressed in this primitive script.

Although the *Neijing Suwen* is the oldest book on Chinese medicine that has come down to us, it seems very unlikely that it was the first book ever to have been written on the subject. Its style does not suggest that it is introducing something new and original. On the contrary, it is clear that by the time it was written, acupuncture was already widely understood and practised in China. In recent times, scholars have suggested that it is, in fact, a compilation of several different treatises, possibly originating from different medical theorists or schools. But there is still no agreement over dating, although many people now believe that the various treatises it comprises were written during a 300 year period between 200 BCE and 100 CE, being put together in one work shortly after this – which, of course, still makes it a work of considerable antiquity.

The *Neijing Suwen* is not a book for beginners – it gives no instructions on basic theory nor on the points and techniques to be used (clearly, it assumes that the reader already knows these) and it covers only the more esoteric aspects of theory, such as *"the transmission of the essence and the transmission of the life-giving principle"* and *"the seasons as patterns of the viscera"*.

It is written in the form of a dialogue, the two participants being Huang Ti (the Yellow Emperor) and Ch'i Po, a Taoist teacher and physician. (In ancient times Chinese physicians were often religious teachers as well, in much the same way that many Western monks were highly skilled in herbal medicine.) The Yellow Emperor asks questions and these are answered at length by Ch'i Po. Some of the questions are very profound, running to several pages, and among the things that Ch'i Po is asked to explain are *"how it is possible that the twelve viscera send each other that which is precious and that which is worthless"* and *"whether the brain and the marrow govern the viscera or whether it is the stomach that governs the viscera, or whether the viscera govern the six bowels"*. The Yellow Emperor – real or mythical – clearly had a very good grasp of the basic theories of Chinese medicine!

BIAN QUE

Further proof of the antiquity of acupuncture comes from stories of the great acupuncturists who lived two thousand or more years ago. Around the fourth century BCE, there was a famous itinerant Chinese physician and teacher of medicine called Bian Que – pronounced Pien Chueh. One story tells of a time when he was visiting the province of Kuo with some of his students or apprentices. Upon reaching the town in which the king and his court resided, they saw that many sacrifices were being offered at the temples and that preparations were being made for a funeral. When Bian Que asked what was happening, he was told that the king's son had suddenly fallen ill and lapsed into a coma from which the court physicians had been unable to rouse him. It seemed inevitable that he would die. Bian Que asked his informant whether he could arrange for him to be introduced at court, since he thought he might be able to prevent the boy from dying. Arrangements were quickly made and the king willingly allowed Bian Que to examine the comatose prince.

After a thorough examination, Bian Que made a diagnosis based on his extensive knowledge of Chinese medicine, and then proceeded to treat the prince with acupuncture, placing needles in his head, chest, arms and legs. Very soon, the boy regained consciousness. Over the next three weeks, Bian Que continued to treat him with acupuncture, heat treatment and herbal remedies, restoring the prince to full health. The story does not tell us what happened to the court physicians, but it is possible that the king made arrangements for them to learn the basics of acupuncture!

MOXA AND MOXIBUSTION

It is likely that the heat treatment that Bian Que used on the prince was moxibustion – a method, still in use today, in which the acupuncture points are warmed in order to stimulate them. The heat comes from burning moxa, which is made from the leaves of the mugwort plant (artemisia vulgaris). The usual practice nowadays is to attach a small wad of moxa to the handle end of the acupuncture needle so that, when it is lit, the heat travels down the needle and into the acupuncture point without running the risk of burning the patient's skin. Originally, however, the custom was to put the moxa directly onto the skin, or onto a slice of ginger placed over the relevant point, and this latter method is still used by some practitioners.

How moxibustion fits into the chronology of acupuncture is uncertain. Some people believe that it may predate acupuncture, since some ancient texts have been found that mention moxa but make no reference to needling. In fact, these particular texts were found in a tomb that dates back to the Han dynasty (206 BCE to 220 CE) – a time during which, as we know from other sources, acupuncture was already being widely used, but they may have been copies of other texts that were considerably older. And, although moxa has been used therapeutically for many centuries, it seems likely that the healing quality of warmth applied to the acupuncture points was known long before the burning properties of moxa leaves were discovered and also before needles were used to treat the points. It is possible that twigs and grass were originally used to produce a similar effect and records show that various other substances, such as charcoal, bamboo and sulphur, have all been used in the past.

The dried moxa leaves, when burned, smell not unlike cannabis – or so I was once told by a teenage patient who informed me that my consulting room smelled like a rock concert! Moxa, like cannabis or that other dried leaf of ill repute, tobacco, has the ability to burn slowly and steadily. It is used primarily to treat diseases said to have been caused by cold or damp (this will be discussed in depth in chapter 4). And although it was, and still is, often found to be useful in its homeland of China, is has been used to a far greater extent in Japan. Being made up of islands, Japan tends to have a much more humid climate than the great expanse of China, so its incidence of diseases associated with damp is much greater. It is therefore appropriate that the name by which this treatment is known in the West – moxa –derives from the Japanese *mo kusa*, meaning 'burning herb'. The Chinese name for moxa is *jiu* which means 'to cauterise' or 'to blister'.

THE ORIGINS OF ACUPUNCTURE

Strangely, in view of China's many ancient myths and folk heroes, there is not, as far as I know, any legend explaining how acupuncture originated. However, it has been suggested that the accidental burning of acupuncture points may have led to the discovery of their therapeutic value. In the days when people huddled around fires that served the dual purpose of keeping them warm and cooking their food, it is likely that they were frequently burned by sparks flying out from the fire. If a spark landed on and burned an appropriate acupuncture point, people may have been 'miraculously' cured of various illnesses that had been troubling them. After this had happened on a number of occasions and to a number of people, the more astute of them may have started to realise that in some way these particular points on the body had healing properties.

Acupuncture points are not scattered randomly over the body but, rather, lie along a well-defined system of meridians or energy channels. In some patients, stimulation of a single point will cause a sensation to run along the meridian on which it lies. In others, needling an individual point may cause a flush to spread along the line of the meridian. Based on this, the early Chinese could have started to work out a system of lines that joined the points together – the predecessors of the meridians that we know today. And, of course, it would appear to them that the way in which to use these points therapeutically was to burn them, since it was through burning that the effects seemed to arise.

Another theory concerning the origin of acupuncture is that, in the days when there was constant warring between neighbouring tribes, men who were wounded in battle may have found that injuries inflicted on certain parts of the body had a therapeutic effect on various diseases from which they were suffering. This is a theory much loved by cartoonists, who depict men lying on the battlefield, run through with spears or stuck full of arrows, making comments such as "That's done wonders for my hay fever".

Other possibilities may seem more feasible. I have heard it suggested that the earliest therapists were healers who used the 'laying on of hands' method which is common all over the world. Healers nowadays often say that they feel a sensation in their hands – cold, heat or tingling – when they have their hands over an area of the patient's body that is in need of treatment. It is possible that these early healers may have been particularly sensitive and intuitive and were thus able to pick up the position of acupuncture points that needed treating, developing the theory of the meridians from there.

According to another theory, the treatment may originally have involved piercing the skin in a fairly random way to drive out devils whose presence in the body was thought to be the cause of illness. Eventually it might have been possible for those performing the treatment to work out which points were effective for which types of illness and, from there, to develop the more elaborate theories of acupuncture.

A fascinating and fairly recent discovery is that the Chinese seem not to have been the only people developing these ideas in the prehistoric period. In 1991, the body of a man was found ten thousand feet up a glacier in the Ötztal Alps on the border between Austria and Italy. Nicknamed "Ötzi", the perfectly preserved body was dated to somewhere between 3350 and 3105 BCE. Various wounds suggested that he had been murdered, and further examination revealed an arthritic condition that would have caused him pain in his back and hips. However, the thing that caught people's attention was the fact that he was covered in tattoos – 61 in total – which seemed to have been created by rubbing fire ash or soot into little incisions or punctures, probably repeatedly. What is more, these tattoos seemed to correspond to acupuncture points and meridians. Acupuncturist Dr Frank Bahr, when asked for his opinion, said that 90 per cent of the points marked by the tattoos would be appropriate for treating a patient with the arthritic problems demonstrated by Ötzi. The tattooing, he suggested, was a prehistoric form of 'doctor's letter' – a message from one practitioner to another indicating which points should be used to treat the patient.

THE TOOLS OF TREATMENT

If it is indeed the case that acupuncture was being used in Europe five thousand years ago, we have an additional conundrum. Not only do we not know how and why acupuncture developed, but we are also unclear why it developed and thrived in China but died out elsewhere. It seems unlikely that we shall ever find out.

What we can be fairly sure of, however, is that once the acupuncture points were discovered – by whatever means – the next stage would have been to experiment with different methods of stimulating them. The earliest acupuncture tools seem to have been sharp pieces of stone or flint (known as bian stones), or sharp pieces of pottery. Their use would have been limited because of their size and shape, so they were probably used just to scratch, or possibly to prick, the points on the meridian.

The next instruments to be developed were somewhat more versatile, being made from sharpened bones or bamboo which could be carved into a more needle-like shape. However, it was not until the smelting of metal had been discovered that it was possible to manufacture true needles that could be inserted through the patient's skin and into the layers below.

The earliest needles were made from various types of metals as they became available – iron, bronze, silver and even gold. Silver and gold acupuncture needles have been found in the tomb of Prince Liu Sheng who died in 113 BCE, suggesting perhaps that the people of the period thought that, even in heaven, their health might need attention!

Since metal was so much more versatile than the stones, bones and bamboo that had previously been used, it became possible to develop different shapes of needles which could then be used for different techniques. These may originally have been made by chance since, presumably, the earliest metal-smithing was a fairly crude affair that could not be expected to produce identical needles every time. Presented with these varying shapes, however, the early acupuncture practitioners may have realised that differently shaped needles produced different effects. So, as the quality of the smithing improved, they would have ordered the specific shapes that they found most useful.

When *The Yellow Emperor's Classic* was compiled some two thousand years ago, nine types of needles were already in common use, not unlike the variety of needles still in use today. There were fine needles which, as now, were used for the majority of treatments. There were arrowhead needles which were used when it was only necessary to prick the point, rather than to insert a needle. To induce slight bleeding at a point, three-sided needles were available. Needles with a triangular tip terminating in a sharp point are still used today when bleeding is required. Blunt or round-ended needles were used when points needed pressure or massaging, and scalpel-like needles were used to incise boils and abscesses. Larger, heavier needles were available for inserting into joints and extra-long needles were used when the most receptive part of the acupuncture point lay well below the skin surface in an area of thick muscle or fat. The longest needles nowadays, used to treat points in areas such as the buttocks, are about three inches long, but much longer ones are believed to have been used by the early acupuncturists.

The majority of needles used in acupuncture practice today are made of stainless steel, which was first developed in the early years of the twentieth century. Although they can be easily sterilised, the appearance of AIDS in the early 1980s and the increase in cases of hepatitis that can be transmitted through blood means that the vast majority of needles which are used nowadays are disposable – used once only and then thrown away.

Before the development of stainless steel, however, silver and gold needles were quite widely used because these two metals are relatively inert and less likely than others to cause unwanted reactions when inserted into the skin. There may have been other reasons for their popularity, too. It was thought that gold needles had, of themselves, a stimulating effect (something that was also said to be true of the other yellow metal, copper), while silver and other white metal needles had a calming effect. Today, needles made of precious metals have definite disadvantages, in that they are much more expensive than stainless steel which means that when they become blunt they have to be resharpened rather than being thrown away. However, they are still used by some practitioners who believe they have intrinsic therapeutic effects. A letter from a Spanish doctor, published in the mid 1980s in the American Journal of Acupuncture, said he had found that, when treating patients for pain, gold needles worked best when the pain was made worse by movement or was due to inflammation and silver worked best for conditions such as repetitive strain injury when the pain had been caused by overuse of the part concerned.

THE TRAINING OF AN ACUPUNCTURIST

In the same way that Western medical students learn both general medicine and surgery as part of their basic curriculum, students in China have always been taught both herbal medicine and acupuncture, both of which are based on the same fundamental theories of body function and energy flow. For centuries, student physicians would train by doing an apprenticeship with an experienced doctor, but in 443 CE the first state-sponsored school in China to teach all aspects of Chinese medicine was opened. However, it closed within ten years and it wasn't until the beginning of the Sui dynasty in 581 CE that an Imperial Medical Academy was founded. But it was only under the following Tang dynasty (618-906) that medical education really became formalised. In 624 CE the academy was greatly enlarged, with departments being set up to teach pharmacology, acupuncture, internal medicine and massage – as well as Buddhist and Taoist incantation which, at the time were thought to be essential knowledge for a physician. For the first time it became possible to study acupuncture and moxibustion as disciplines in their own right, separate from herbal medicine.

The length of training required to become a physician was as long as, or longer than, that required in the West today. Before a student was allowed to specialise in any one aspect of medicine, he had to take a general introductory course. Once he had passed this, he was allowed to study internal medicine (which took a further seven years), or surgery (which took five years) or paediatrics (which also took five years). Less time was needed to train in more limited specialities such as diseases of the ear, nose and throat.

Like medical schools today, the Imperial Medical Academy taught from standard textbooks. *The Yellow Emperor's Classic* was, of course, one of them. Another was Huang-fu Mi's *Classic of Acupuncture and Moxibustion* (*Zhenjiu Jiayi Jing*), written in the third century CE and the oldest known book that is devoted entirely to acupuncture and moxibustion. Many later books used this book as a source, and it played an important role in the development of acupuncture in Japan and Korea. A third standard text in use at the Imperial Medical Academy was Wang Shu-he's *Classic of the Pulse* (*Mai Jing*).

THE FOUR TECHNIQUES OF DIAGNOSIS

Bian Que is said to have been the first physician to use all the four basic techniques of Chinese diagnosis. The first of these is observation, in which the physician notes the patient's facial expression and observes his complexion, colour, skin and tongue in much the same way that a Western doctor does today – although, of course, these findings would be interpreted differently by the Chinese physician. The tongue, like the pulse, can tell a traditionally trained Chinese physician far more than it can tell a Western doctor, and its observation is an important method of diagnosis. (This, too, will be described more fully in chapter 5.)

The second technique, or group of techniques, used by Bian Que comprised listening and smelling. He would listen to the quality of the patient's speech – normal, slurred, high pitched and so on – and to the sound of his breathing although, of course, he lacked the benefit of that modern Western tool, the stethoscope. He would also smell the patient's body odours – probably more important in a society where hot and cold running water were unknown and baths were likely to have been taken only infrequently. The noting of bodily smells is still used by acupuncturists using the Five Elements system (see chapter 3) and can even be of use, on occasion, in modern Western medicine. For example, the smell of acetone on a patient's breath can be an indication that she is a diabetic whose condition is getting out of control.

The third technique on Bian Que's list was questioning which, of course, plays an important role in all forms of medicine – Western, Chinese and other complementary therapies. And, finally, he would use pulse diagnosis.

Pulse taking (which will be discussed in some depth in chapter 5) is a much more exact and detailed science in Chinese medicine than it is in the West, and it plays a far more important role in diagnosis. It can take a student many years to become an expert in interpreting the pulse. And, because not just acupuncture but all forms of traditional Chinese medicine are based on the same theories of the causation of disease, pulse diagnosis is fundamental to all of them.

When Wang Shu-he wrote *The Classic of the Pulse*, he was not expounding a newly developed science but, rather, was producing a compendium of ancient diagnostic techniques that had grown up alongside Chinese medicine as it developed. Other books, published long before *The Classic of the Pulse*, had mentioned pulse diagnosis – in fact, the oldest of them all, *The Yellow Emperor's Classic*, gives some quite detailed descriptions of the quality of the pulse in different disease states. The great acupuncturist Bian Que, whom we have already met in the story of his treatment of the comatose prince of Kuo, is known to have used pulse diagnosis. And it was, no doubt, his ability as a diagnostician in addition to his skills in treatment, that enabled him to treat the prince successfully when the court physicians had failed.

SPREAD TO OTHER COUNTRIES

The Classic of the Pulse was exported to Japan and Korea in the sixth century CE. Chinese medicine had reached both countries several centuries earlier and techniques of pulse diagnosis were rapidly assimilated into their medical practice. *The General Treatise on Causes and Manifestations of All Diseases* (*Zhubing Yuanhou Lun*) published only a few years later, in 610 CE, was also to become extremely influential in the development of Japanese and Korean medicine. Its grandiose title was perhaps justified since it stretched to fifty volumes and contained virtually all the medical knowledge of the time. Its editor was Chao Yuanfang, a physician at the Imperial court.

As Chinese medicine developed during the Tang dynasty (618-906), its fame spread. Soon physicians from other countries were arriving in China to learn new techniques. These included Arabian doctors who came to learn the art of pulse diagnosis and to study infectious diseases. *The Classic of the Pulse* was exported to the Middle East some time in the eleventh century and, by the mid-fourteenth century, had been translated into Turkish. The great Persian physician Abu-Ali al-Husain ibn Abdullah ibn Sina, better known as Avicenna (980-1037) wrote an immense work in Arabic called *The Canon of Medicine* (*Al-Qanun f'il-Tibb*) in which he discussed the medical achievements of the great Greek physicians and described medical techniques that had been written about in other Arabic works. To this he added information about the methods that he himself had developed during his own years of practice, based on what he had been taught during his travels and what he had learned from reading. Among these was pulse diagnosis, and he recorded twenty four different types of pulse of which he was aware.

REVISION AND DEVELOPMENT

Meanwhile, in China during the Song dynasty (960-1279), acupuncture and moxibustion became very popular, mainly due to the patronage of the Imperial court and the nobility. And acupuncture and the diagnostic techniques of Chinese medicine were now becoming familiar in other parts of Asia and in the Middle East. But, despite all this – or perhaps because of it – the Chinese Imperial court was concerned that, over the years, inaccuracies had arisen in the practice of the therapy. Many of the early books on acupuncture had been lost and many of the standard reference books were compilations into which errors could easily have crept. As a result of this concern, the court turned to Wang Weiyi who was physician to Emperor Renzong (1022–63) of the Northern Song dynasty. Wang Weiyi was instructed to investigate the validity of the system of acupuncture that was currently being practised and to carry out what would be the first major revision of acupuncture theory.

He embarked on a mammoth research programme, investigating all the acupuncture points that were currently being used and verifying their locations. He also studied each point in turn and confirmed the depth to which each should be punctured in order to produce an effect. Finally, he identified the effects that might be produced by the needling of each point. He published his findings in a work entitled *An Illustrated Manual of Acupuncture Points* (*Tongren Shuxue Zhenjiu Tujing*).

The contribution that Wang Weiyi made to the development of acupuncture and to its teaching was to have long-lasting results. Under the Imperial patronage, he supervised the manufacture of a model of a man, cast in bronze, with the surface punctured with holes accurately placed at the positions of all the acupuncture points. These bronze men became valuable teaching aids and were also used to test the knowledge of students in examinations held at the Imperial Medical Academy. The model would be coated with a thick layer of wax which was allowed to set so that the holes could not be seen. The hollow interior of the model was then filled with water. The student would be given a case history and asked how he would use acupuncture to treat the patient. He was expected to name the points he would use, explain why he would use them, and then locate them on the model, inserting a needle into each, through the wax. If he located the points accurately, the needles would go through the wax into the holes beneath so that, when they were removed, water would flow out – and the student would pass his examination.

It may have been his work with these models and with teaching that caused Wang Weiyi's absence from court when his patron, Emperor Renzong, was taken ill in 1034. The Imperial physicians treated the Emperor with methods other than acupuncture, but without success. Eventually, a highly skilled acupuncturist named Xu Xi stepped in and cured him. However, the courtiers in attendance on the Emperor nearly stopped the treatment from taking place. Having examined the patient, Xu Xi let it be known that he would be inserting acupuncture needles into the Emperor's chest, just below the level of his heart. The courtiers were horrified, believing that, far from curing the Emperor, this treatment was likely to kill him. Xu Xi assured them that, on the contrary, the treatment was perfectly safe, and he offered to demonstrate the technique on someone whose death, if it occurred, would be less of a disaster. The courtiers agreed to this and told Xu Xi that he could demonstrate the technique on the court eunuchs who, presumably, were expendable. Needles were inserted at the points that Xu Xi had described and the courtiers were amazed and relieved to find that he had spoken the truth – the eunuchs were unharmed. (No doubt the eunuchs were even more relieved!) Xu Xi lost no time in treating the Emperor who then made a rapid recovery and rewarded Xu Xi by appointing him medical officer to the Imperial Medical Academy.

Wang Weiyi's bronze models continued to be used for the next five hundred years but, in the mid-sixteenth century, they were taken a step further by an acupuncturist named Kao Wu. Concerned that all these models were of men, and aware that the location of acupuncture points differed according to the sex and the age of the patient, he arranged to have bronze figures cast of women and children. He also wrote two important books – *Essentials of Acupuncture and Moxibustion*, a summary of earlier major works which was intended for new students, and *Eminent Acupuncture* for more advanced students and qualified practitioners.

Around this time, many other books were being written that simply revised and summarised the works of earlier authors. However, in 1601, eighty year old acupuncturist Yang Jizhou published *A Compendium of Acupuncture and Moxibustion*. This ten volume work summarises what had been written about acupuncture in previous centuries and also includes a large amount of information based on the results of the author's own research and experience. It was a great success both in China and in the Asian countries to which the practice of acupuncture had spread, and is still in print today.

ACUPUNCTURE AND BUDDHISM

By this time, acupuncture and traditional Chinese medicine were being used far beyond the borders of China. In some countries, such as Japan and Korea, they had become the primary form of medical treatment. Traditional Chinese medicine had first been introduced into these two countries many centuries before, during the Qin Dynasty (221-206 BCE), but it was with the spread of Buddhism that it really began to gain popularity. Buddhism, which originated in India in the sixth century BCE, reached China some time around the middle of the first century CE. There it developed in tradition and practice and, in the second half of the fourth century, was introduced into Korea. Some two hundred years later, it spread to Japan where the Zen school (which today has followers all around the world) developed. Although Buddhism was not an immediate success among the Japanese people, the regent Shotoku Taishi (573-621) was converted and began to encourage Buddhist monks to come to Japan from China.

In China, traditional Chinese medicine and acupuncture often formed part of the studies of Buddhist monks. During the Sui dynasty (581-618) and the Tang dynasty (618-906), many of these physician-monks came to Japan. While they were there, they taught the Japanese people whatever they wanted to learn – not just Buddhist doctrine but also the fundamentals of Chinese medicine.

The earliest Buddhist texts were written in Pali but, with the spread of the religion, more scriptures were written in Sanskrit and in Chinese, and earlier works were translated. However, it took time for these translations to be prepared for a newly converted country, so the texts used by the monks who went to Japan were in Chinese. If the Japanese converts wanted to read the original scriptures and not just hear about them from the monks (who, no doubt, were adding their own interpretations to them) they would have to learn to read Chinese. And this is what many of them did. During the seventh century, young Japanese men started to go to China to learn the language – and many came back with a knowledge not just of the language and of Buddhist scriptures but also of Chinese medicine and acupuncture.

ACUPUNCTURE IN JAPAN

Once enough Japanese physicians were fluent in the Chinese language, translations could be made of the major Chinese medical texts so that they would be available to all. *The Yellow Emperor's Classic* was one of the first to be translated and, by the start of the eighth century, was one of the standard textbooks for Japanese medical students. Large numbers of Chinese medical texts were brought to Japan in the mid-eighth century by the physician and philanthropist Chien Chen who established a charity clinic where the poor could be treated. Centuries later, his work with the sick and needy was still remembered and his name venerated in Japanese temples.

Chinese medicine remained popular in Japan until the sixteenth century when it became overshadowed by influences from the West. This was the period of the great trading companies, with ships being sent from Europe to build up markets and find suppliers of luxuries in far-flung places around the world. The Portuguese, after establishing a foothold in the Far East, sent a number of Roman Catholic missionaries to both China and Japan. Like the Buddhist monks who had come to Japan a thousand years earlier, these missionaries had some knowledge of medicine – although this was, of course, the comparatively primitive medicine being practised in Europe at the time. But, either because it was new and different or perhaps because of the forceful personalities of those who brought it to the East, it usurped the practice of traditional Chinese medicine in Japan.

Over the next three centuries, acupuncture and Chinese medicine were still practised in Japan, but they played second fiddle to Western medicine. In 1884 an attempt was made to wipe them out completely when an edict prohibiting the teaching of acupuncture and herbal medicine anywhere in the country was issued to coincide with the founding of the medical faculty at Tokyo University. Not even this, however, could stop people from practising therapies which they knew to be valuable, and traditional medicine and acupuncture have continued to be used alongside Western techniques up to the present day.

FURTHER DEVELOPMENT IN CHINA

Surprisingly, in 1822 – sixty two years before the teaching of acupuncture and Chinese medicine was prohibited in Japan – their use was banned in China by Emperor Daoguang. The subjects were removed from the syllabus of the Imperial Medical Academy but, as was to happen later in Japan, their use could not be stopped, since the people were aware of their value and would not give them up.

In 1912 the Imperial Qing dynasty was overthrown and replaced by the radical Kuomintang party who ruled China until the end of the Second World War when they, in turn, were ousted by the Communists. The latter, aware of the people's views on acupuncture and traditional Chinese medicine, removed the prohibitions on their use and, for the first time in over a hundred years, treatment with acupuncture was actively encouraged. Many of the ancient Chinese medical books that had been used over the centuries as standard texts were reprinted and many new books were written. Colleges specialising in the teaching of traditional Chinese medicine were set up, all with separate departments for acupuncture. Research institutes were founded for the investigation of acupuncture and the furtherance of its practice. The existing medical schools which, since the ban of 1822, had taught only Western medicine, now put acupuncture back onto the curriculum. Nowadays China has many medical schools and, since 1949, acupuncture has been taught in all of them in an integrated course alongside Western medicine.

Acupuncture also remains popular in a number of other Asian countries. In Vietnam, where it was introduced during the Han dynasty, it became customary in the latter half of the twentieth century for patients who were admitted to hospital to be treated using Western techniques but for acupuncture and traditional herbal medicine to be used for everyday ills.

ACUPUNCTURE IN EUROPE

Until about the start of the twentieth century Western medicine was a fairly crude discipline with little to offer in the way of curative techniques, so it is perhaps surprising that it should so easily have superseded the practice of the far more sophisticated Chinese medicine and acupuncture in the Far East, particularly in Japan and China. Maybe it says something about the willingness of the Chinese and Japanese people to accept new ideas compared with people in the West. By contrast, although acupuncture was introduced into Europe during the seventeenth century, at roughly the same time that Western medicine was having such an impact in the East, it did not become popular among Westerners until the second half of the twentieth century. One possible reason may be that Western medicine, when introduced to the East, was still in its infancy enabling the Chinese and Japanese to learn about it as it developed, but acupuncture was already a highly developed therapy and (to the Western mind) very hard to understand by the time it was introduced into Europe.

On Indian medicine (*De medicina Indorum*), written by the Danish physician and pioneer of tropical medicine Jacob de Bondt, and published in 1631, was probably the first European book to mention acupuncture. However, this was only a passing reference and it was several decades before a book was published which was specifically about Chinese medicine. One of the earliest was by a Jesuit priest, Father Placide Harvieu, and was splendidly entitled *The Secrets of Chinese Medicine and the Perfect Knowledge of the Pulse, Brought from China by a Respected Frenchman*.

In 1682, Andreas Cleyer published his *Examples of Chinese Medicine* (*Specimen Medicinae Sinicae*). Cleyer, a German, was chief commissioner of the Dutch East India Company's colony in Java and had been interested in Chinese medicine since the late 1660s. However, it is not clear how much of the book was his own work and how much was taken from the writings of other people with similar interests. But it was the first illustrated book on Chinese medicine to be published in Europe, and was a major step forward in the understanding of the subject.

Cleyer was helped to compile his book by the Dutch physician and botanist Willem Ten Rhijne who, in 1683, published his own collection of treatises, one of which, for the first time, offered European readers a detailed description of acupuncture therapy and moxibustion, with illustrations of the acupuncture points. This treatise was entitled *About Acupuncture* (*De acupunctura*), the word acupuncture having been coined by Ten Rhijne from the Latin words for 'puncture' and 'needle'.

A quarter of a century later, in 1707, the English physician Sir John Floyer (1649-1734), who had been impressed by Chinese diagnostic techniques, published *The Physician's Pulse-Watch*. In this, he reviewed the old ways in which the pulse had been used in medicine, suggested new methods and, in the third part of the work, wrote about the Chinese art of feeling the pulse and recommended *"the imitation of their practice of physic, which is grounded on the observation of the pulse"*.

It would be another few decades before anyone in the West actually practised the art of acupuncture. The first to do so was probably a French physician, Dr Louis-Joseph Berlioz (1776-1848) who, in 1816, published a book, *Memoirs on Chronic Complaints, Blood-letting and Acupuncture* (*Mémoires sur les maladies chroniques, les évacuations sanguines et l'acupuncture*). Sadly, his pioneering work is scarcely remembered, and the name of Berlioz is associated in most people's minds only with his son, the composer Hector Berlioz.

In the decade following the publication of Dr Berlioz' book, several more on the subject were published in France. In 1825, Dr. J. Morand published *Memoir on Acupuncture, Followed by a Series of Personal Observations Made by Mr. Jules Cloquet* (*Mémoire sur l'Acupuncture, Suivi d'une Série d'Observations Recueillies sous les Yeux de M. Jules Cloquet*) and *A Dissertation on Acupuncture and its Therapeutic Effects* (*Dissertation sur l'acupuncture et ses effets thérapeutiques*). In the same year, the Chevalier Jean Baptiste Sarlandiere (1787-1838) published *Memoirs on Electropuncture, Considered as a New Way to Treat Gout, Rheumatism and Nervous Complaints Effectively, and on the Use of Japanese Moxa in France* (*Mémoires sur l'Électro-puncture, Considérée*

Comme Moyen Nouveau de Traiter Efficacement la Goutte, les Rhumatismes et les Affections Nerveuses, et sur l'Emploi du Moxa Japonais en France). And in 1826 Dr. Jules Cloquet (1790-1883), whose observations had already been published by Dr. Morand, produced his own book, *Treatise on Acupuncture* (*Traité de l'Acupuncture*).

Meanwhile, in London in 1821, James Morss Churchill (who is known primarily as a botanist) published *A Treatise on Acupuncturation*, in which he writes:

> *"It is a little strange that the surprising efficacy of which so much has been boasted by its eastern professors, and the safety, at least, with which acupuncturation may be performed having been so fully demonstrated ... that it has not met with an earlier encouragement amongst us... There have not, however, been wanting sensible minds and men of talent and reputation to recommend this operation; and the names of Ten-Rhyne, Bidloo, Koempfer and Vicq-d'Azyr stand conspicuous on the list of those who speak in its favour; but still, none of them had undertaken to put its merits to the test by actual experiment. Several practitioners in France, however, have now taken up this neglected operation and their report verifies the praises which have been bestowed by others upon it. My attention was lately directed to it by my friend Mr Scott, of Westminster, who, as far as my knowledge goes, was the first who performed it in England, and some successful cases which I witnessed in his practice assured me of its efficacy and led me to its adoption. The success of my own subsequent practice warrants a recommendation of it in almost any terms I could give it."*

Of the five names mentioned by Churchill, we have already met Willem Ten-Rhyne. Koempfer refers to the German naturalist and physician Englelbert Kaempfer (1651-1716) who had become interested in acupuncture and moxibustion while in Japan and subsequently wrote an influential treatise *An Account of the Moxa, an Excellent Caustic of the Chinese and Japanese, with a Scheme Shewing What Parts of the Human Body Are to be Burnt With That Plant in Several Distempers* which was included as an appendix in his three volume work *A History of Japan*. Felix Vicq d'Azyr (1748-1794) was a French anatomist who had the dubious distinction of being Queen Marie Antoinette's physician and was possibly the very first French author to mention acupuncture in his writings. Bidloo refers either to Govert Bidloo (1649-1713), a Dutch anatomist, or his nephew Nicolaas Bidloo (1674-1735) who was the personal physician of Peter the Great of Russia – but the connection of either man to acupuncture is hard to ascertain. As to Mr. Scott of Westminster – sadly, his identity is lost in the mists of time.

French physicians continued to be interested in acupuncture. In the early 20th century Georges Soulie de Morant, the representative of a French bank who lived in China for over 20 years and eventually became French consul, trained in acupuncture and was awarded the title of Master Physician. He translated several works on Chinese medicine and wrote two books of his own: *The Synopsis of the True Chinese Acupuncture* (published in 1934) and the two-volume *Acupuncture*, published in 1939.

Meanwhile, in Germany, the establishment of a Chinese medicine research institute in 1906 sparked off the publication of many new books on traditional Chinese medicine and acupuncture.

It was not until the mid 20th century, however, that acupuncture started to be noticed and investigated in Britain. In 1957 Dr Louis Moss, a London general practitioner, wrote to *The Lancet* about the treatment of some two thousand patients with arthritis using 'trigger points' which seemed to tally with certain acupuncture points and which had given permanent relief from pain. The following year a group of British doctors went to Germany to investigate the use of acupuncture and shortly after that, in 1959, Dr Felix Mann founded the Medical Acupuncture Society (later the British Medical Acupuncture Society).

ACUPUNCTURE IN NORTH AMERICA

In the United States and Canada, acupuncture and traditional Chinese medicine was brought by the Chinese people who settled there from the early 19th century onwards. But these people, together with their customs and therapies, tended to remain within their own communities. There was some outside interest in the subject but it was very sporadic.

The person credited with introducing acupuncture to the American medical profession was Dr. Franklin Baché (a great-grandson of Benjamin Franklin) who, in 1825, published a translation of Dr. Morand's *Memoir on Acupuncture*. In his introduction to the book, Baché wrote

> *"The original of the present Memoir was put into my hands by my friend, Dr. Samuel Brown . . . with a request that I would prepare a translation of it for the American medical public. I readily acceded to his wishes, believing, with him, that a short treatise on Acupuncturation, from the growing importance of the remedy, and the great attention bestowed upon it in France, could not fail to be an acceptable present to American physicians. The present Memoir, after an historical introduction, proceeds to give an account of the manner of using the needle, and concludes with a number of cases, illustrative of its effects. Without going too much into detail, it imparts every requisite information, to enable any practitioner to employ the remedy."*

This last claim was somewhat far-fetched, since the memoir, while going into great detail about the needles themselves and the effects of inserting them into both people and animals, contains nothing whatsoever about the theory of acupuncture or the location of the acupuncture points.

Maybe it was because of this deficiency that the book failed to arouse the interest that Baché had hoped for. A decade later, in 1836, two articles by Dr William Markley Lee were published recommending acupuncture for pain relief and as a "remedy for rheumatism". But after this there was very little until the publication of *The Chinese Way of Medicine* by Edward Hume in 1940 and a partial translation of *The Yellow Emperor's Classic* by Ilza Veith in 1949. However, although Dr Veith's familiarity with the Chinese language allowed her to produce a readable and informative translation of this very difficult work, it is obvious that she had had no personal experience of acupuncture when she started work on the book. In the introduction she wrote *"The practice of acupuncture and moxibustion has survived, despite the fact that these treatments must be exceedingly painful to the patient"* – a clear indication that she had never even seen a patient being treated with acupuncture, let alone experienced it. In fact, in the preface to the revised 1965 edition of the book, she wrote that when she did the original translation *"the subject of my study seemed to be entirely esoteric"*.

ACUPUNCTURE AS AN ANAESTHETIC

The realisation that acupuncture could be used in place of anaesthesia to control pain during operations was a major step forward. Its effectiveness in relieving pain caused by disease had, of course, been known for centuries in the countries where it was practised. However, surgery only started to be performed on a large scale at the end of the 19th century and it wasn't until 1958 that Chinese doctors started to use acupuncture to control postoperative pain. The results they obtained were so good that they decided to see whether it was possible to control the pain of a minor operation – tonsillectomy was the first to be tried – without having to use any other form of anaesthesia. Again, the results were excellent so doctors started to use acupuncture for other minor operations such as tooth extractions and the repair of hernias. Although they found that not all patients treated with acupuncture developed a sufficient degree of anaesthesia to allow it to be used as the sole method of pain control during an operation, many patients were able to tolerate surgery without any other form of anaesthetic.

FINAL ACCEPTANCE OF ACUPUNCTURE IN THE WEST

It was this step forward plus President Nixon's visit to China in 1972 that finally brought acupuncture to the public's attention in the West. President Nixon's personal physician, Dr Walter R. Tkach, accompanied him to China and was invited to visit Friendship Hospital in Beijing where he watched three operations being performed – to remove a thyroid cyst, a cataract and an ovarian cyst – all under acupuncture anaesthesia. And on his return to the USA, he wrote an article for the *Readers Digest* entitled *I Watched Acupuncture Work*.

Since the 1970s acupuncture has grown enormously in popularity in the West. There are some 5,000 registered acupuncturists in the UK and nearly 40,000 in the USA. In 2018, American colleges and universities were offering 32 Masters degrees in acupuncture and 53 in oriental medicine. In the UK there are seven accredited specialist colleges offering licentiates or Bachelor degrees in acupuncture and Chinese medicine. Many thousands of patients every year are realising the benefits of this therapy. Acupuncture is here to stay.

2

FUNDAMENTAL PRINCIPLES

HOLISM AND HOLISTIC THERAPIES

Acupuncture is often referred to as a holistic therapy. The word *holism* seems to have been coined in the 1920s by the South African statesman Jan Smuts and is defined by the Oxford English Dictionary as *"the tendency in nature to produce wholes from the ordered grouping of units"*. (Sometimes you will see it spelled *wholism* although Smuts derived it from the Greek word *holos* – meaning '*whole*' – and not from the English word *whole*.)

Although they are often used interchangeably when describing a therapy, *holistic* is not synonymous with *complementary* or *alternative*. A holistic therapy is one that treats the patient as a whole. And, although most complementary therapies are holistic when properly used, it is perfectly possible to use most, if not all, of them in a non-holistic way.

Equally, because much of holism resides in the attitude of the therapist towards the patient, it is perfectly possible for a practitioner of orthodox Western medicine to work holistically by taking account of all the patient's problems and relating them to the patient as a whole. Indeed, this was the strength of the old-fashioned family doctor, compared with today's overworked general practitioner. The family doctor knew each of his patients individually; he knew their parents, their husbands or wives, and their children, because all of them would have been his patients too. He knew where his patients worked, the sort of food that they could afford, and the kind of housing they lived in. He was a part of the community, living in the same town or village as his patients, and he got to know many of them socially. When he made a house call to visit one patient, he would probably be given a chance to speak to other members of the family, many of whom would be living nearby. It was therefore a great deal easier for him to see the patient as a whole than it is for today's general practitioner whose patients may well live some distance from the rest of their family, whose backgrounds and places of work he does not know, who may have become his patients only in adult life, and whose previous medical notes he doesn't have time to read.

However, it is not just today's larger and more mobile populations that prevent orthodox doctors from practising holistically. Western medicine's dependence on the use of drugs and of surgery makes it impossible for it to be holistic therapy. Surgery, of course, cannot be holistic since it is based on the principle that if a part of the patient is diseased, that part needs to be removed or replaced or repaired. Modern drugs, too, are formulated to have a specific action on only one or two particular conditions. So, for example, we have anti-arthritic drugs, hypotensive drugs (to reduce the blood pressure), tranquilisers, antibiotics, sleeping pills, and pain killers. By contrast, a holistic therapy such as acupuncture or homoeopathy has to relate to all aspects of the patient, and not just to the symptoms that are being experienced, in order to produce the best results.

So patients receiving orthodox treatment for several complaints tend to have to take a number of different tablets to control them all. But if a patient is suffering from, say, bronchitis, arthritis and high blood pressure, a holistic therapy used correctly may well produce an improvement in all three conditions, since its action is to raise the level of health of the whole patient, allowing the body to fight back against all the problems that are afflicting it. There is no way that a Western practitioner can prescribe a single medication that will do this, no matter how much he might wish to. Nor has any orthodox drug been found that can raise a patient's entire level of health. But this sort of treatment is quite possible for a truly holistic therapy.

The point about a holistic therapy is that it does not treat a single symptom or even a single disease. It treats the patient. And each patient is an individual unlike any other, a fact that Western doctors are also well aware of. The controlled trials that are used in Western medicine to compare two forms of treatment, or to establish the efficacy of a new treatment, involve using two comparable groups of patients. And it is not always easy to find enough 'matched' patients, even when the matching criteria are as basic as age, sex, and the length of time that the patient has been ill. Think how much harder it would be to match patients if you also had to include things such as weight, temperament, marital status, number of children, job, level of education, financial status, housing and so on. And yet all these things contribute to that patient being the person he is.

In a holistic therapy, then, every patient is treated individually because what relieves the symptoms of one may have no effect at all on another who, in orthodox terms, appears to have the same complaint. Even in Western medicine it is acknowledged that two patients given the same drug may react quite differently to it. Not all patients with arthritis, for example, can be treated with the same medication – some will find it helpful, but others will show little response or will develop side effects whose severity outweighs the relief obtained from taking the drug. And this is one reason why a large number of drugs may be available for the treatment of a single condition. Most doctors have their favourite drugs for common conditions – those that seem to them to be most effective and that they will always use as their first choice. But trying to find the right medication for a patient always has something of a hit-and-miss aspect to it, simply because a doctor can never tell in advance exactly how this patient, as opposed to the last patient or the next one, will respond to this particular drug.

In acupuncture, however, the system of diagnosis is geared to finding an individual tailor-made treatment for an individual patient. In Western medicine, a diagnosis – and therefore the treatment prescribed – is based on determining which particular organ, system or part is malfunctioning. And the diagnosis is made in terms relating to that part, such as heart attack, gallbladder disease, kidney stones, nasal polyps, varicose veins and so on. In other words, the diagnosis is usually a description of the end result of the disease process. It is not related to any causative factors. This is not to say that Western medicine is not interested in preventive medicine, but the emphasis in disease remains firmly on the disease process and its end result.

Prevention, however, can be undertaken on various levels. For instance, there are three ways to prevent infection. The first is to give the patient a prophylactic antibiotic so that if her system is invaded by bacteria, the antibiotic will kill them and she will not become ill. This is frequently used for patients with recurrent urinary tract infections. However, the major drawback of this is that taking the antibiotic long term may result in bacteria becoming resistant to it. The second way to prevent infection is to examine the environment, find out where the bacteria are coming from, and eradicate them. This is the way in which most orthodox prevention works and most British doctors know the story of the Broad Street pump – when, in 1854, Dr. John Snow removed the handle from the pump in London's Soho to try to prevent people from drinking contaminated water that he believed was the cause of a serious outbreak of cholera.

The third method of prevention, however, is the holistic way – treating the patient as a whole so that his own natural defences are strong enough to resist any attack that may occur. And this is the basis on which patients are treated by acupuncture. The focus is on energies and the diagnosis is concerned with how these bodily energies are malfunctioning rather than with the manifestations of disease that a particular malfunction has caused. The area in which the disease appears (such as the heart, gallbladder, or kidney) is merely an indication of how the body has been affected by the disruption of its energies. In other words, heart disease does not mean that there is a problem heart in an otherwise healthy body, or even that the heart itself needs to be treated. What it does mean is that the patient's vital energies have become disrupted in a way that has manifested as disease of the heart. The disease manifestation is a clue to the acupuncturist as to how to treat the patient in order to restore her to health, but it is nothing more.

Here, then, is the basic difference between Western drug therapy and acupuncture. A patient who is prescribed drugs for his condition may be lucky the first time – many are – and rapidly obtain relief. However, others will have to try a succession of possible treatments before they see any worthwhile improvement in their condition, and they may have to put up with unpleasant side effects along the way. But a patient being treated by an expert acupuncturist who makes a correct holistic diagnosis will be given a treatment that is tailored to her needs from the very beginning. Another major difference is that in many cases of chronic illness, such as arthritis, chronic bronchitis, or psoriasis, the patient who is treated by Western means may have to remain on medication for life, since the drugs, although possibly controlling the symptoms admirably, may have no effect on the underlying condition. Because acupuncture and other holistic therapies treat the body in such a way as to raise it to a level of energy at which it can heal itself, they may be able to reverse chronic diseases to a certain extent. After a successful course of treatment it may be months or even years before the patient needs to see his practitioner again.

It must be said, of course, that not every patient will respond to acupuncture, even in expert hands. Here again, the patient is an individual. In the same way that there is no one drug that suits every patient, there is no one therapy that suits everyone. Indeed, for those patients who respond well to Western therapy and experience no unpleasant side effects, there would seem to be no advantage in looking elsewhere, because sometimes people have to try more than one complementary therapy before finding the one that works for them.

QI

The Chinese see the whole functioning of the body and mind as being dependent on the normal flow of body energies or life force, which they call *qi* (pronounced 'chee')

But *qi* is not just the life force of the individual person or animal, and my *qi* is not distinct from your *qi*. *Qi* is a universal energy that surrounds and pervades everything, both animate and inanimate. Like radio waves or ultraviolet light, we cannot see *qi* or feel it – we can only recognise it in terms of its effects. Radio waves, when picked up by a receiver tuned to the right frequency, will transmit sound. But a radio through which radio waves do not pass cannot itself produce any sounds. In the same way, *qi* is apparent to us as the life force of a body, and a body that no longer has *qi* circulating through it is dead. But, in the same way that radio waves do not depend on radio sets for their existence and therefore do not disappear when a set is broken, so the *qi* that permeates a body does not just disappear at its death. *Qi* is in a constant state of flux; there is constant interchange between the *qi* of the body and the *qi* of the environment, or external *qi*. And in the same way that food can be good or bad, nourishing or poisonous, external *qi* can also be good or harmful.

Like air and food, *qi* is taken in from the outside in the processes of breathing and eating. This external *qi* is transformed within the body and used to replenish the internal *qi*. Waste *qi* is eliminated in the same way as the end products of respiration and digestion. Within the body *qi* performs several specific functions, one of which is to form protective *qi*. If this protective *qi* is strong, it acts as a defence against any harmful external *qi* with which you may come into contact. If your protective *qi* is weak, however, your resistance is lowered and you can be attacked by harmful external *qi*. If this happens, the body becomes ill. This is a concept that is also understood, although in different terms, in Western medicine. Most people are aware that if they are stressed or overtired, or if their diet is poor, they are more likely to suffer from infections. What a nutritionist would call nutrient-rich food might be referred to by a Chinese physician as food rich in *qi*. This interesting analogy can, to a certain extent, be demonstrated physically by Kirlian electrography, a method in which an image is obtained on photographic paper of the energy (or corona discharge) emanating from a person or object. Its main use is as a diagnostic tool and an adjunct to complementary therapies, when pictures taken of a patient's hands and feet can point to abnormalities in the body's energy field. Pictures can also be obtained of inanimate objects. It has been found that foods high in nutritional value, such as green vegetables and whole-grain bread, have a much better corona discharge than junk foods that contain few vitamins or minerals. Whether what the pictures show as a corona discharge is what the Chinese know as *qi* has not yet been proved, but there is no doubt that when we eat nutritionally wholesome food, we are also ingesting some form of energy.

Thus the patient on a poor diet may be opening herself to attack by lowering her defences. Stress, too, can break down our resistance to illness. Chinese medical theory recognises that not all disease comes from outside as an attack by harmful *qi*; it may also be due to imbalances arising within, often as a result of emotional problems.

Whether or not we get ill depends not just on the viruses, bacteria, carcinogens and other outside influences waiting to attack us but also, and more importantly, on our own inner resistance or protective *qi*. This idea is not alien to the thinking of Western physicians – although, of course, they express it in different terms. In his book *Cancer and Its Nutritional Therapies* (Keats Publishing, 1986) Dr Richard Passwater commented that *"fanatical avoidance of every possible carcinogen is not possible. They are everywhere . . . The best hope remains in always retaining a strong immune response"*.

Whether we are thinking in terms of *qi* or of immune response, once we have become ill, our inner resistance is also of vital importance in determining how easily and quickly we get better. By raising our level of health, the therapist can reinforce our intrinsic resistance to disease, and thus we can be helped to heal ourselves.

Some people, of course, just never seem to get ill, whereas others are laid low by every bug that goes around. This is beautifully illustrated by a scene in Billy Wilder's film *The Apartment*. The hero, C.C. Baxter (played by Jack Lemmon) catches a streaming cold after he has been shut out of his apartment in pouring rain for the best part of the night. The next morning he steps into the elevator at the New York insurance company where he works and tells Fran Kubelik, the elevator operator (Shirley MacLaine) not to stand too close for fear of catching his germs.

"I never get colds," she says casually. Baxter is impressed. He tells her that he has been examining the statistics on colds and asks, "Did you know that the average New Yorker between twenty and fifty has two and a half colds a year?"

"That makes me feel just terrible," says Fran.

"Why?" asks Baxter.

"Well, to make the figures come out even, if I have no colds a year, some poor slob must have five colds a year."

"Yes," agrees Baxter, "It's me."

In Chinese terms, people such as C.C. Baxter are out of balance, whereas Fran Kubelik and others like her are in balance. If Fran had stayed out all night in the rain, she probably wouldn't have caught a cold. At most she might have developed just a temporary sniffle. People like this have strong protective *qi*. They are taking in plenty of good qi to replenish their internal *qi*. And *qi* is circulating around their bodies normally, not encountering any blockages and enjoying perfect balance between its opposing negative and positive aspects, *yin* and *yang*.

YIN AND YANG

Like *qi*, *yin* and *yang* pervade everything. However, unlike *qi*, they are not energies in themselves but, rather, aspects of everything, each being unable to exist without the other. You can think of them in the same terms as right and left: neither can be described without reference to the other, and yet, as a pair, they are totally understandable and useful concepts. *Yin* and *yang* have their own individual qualities and, because these qualities are the opposite of each other, *yin* and *yang* must be in perfect balance within the body in order to maintain perfect health. An imbalance will cause malfunction in the same way that an object that is much larger and heavier on its right side than on its left may well topple over.

Yin pertains to coldness, slowness, dimness, quietness, and solidity, and is associated with female characteristics and the night. *Yang*, on the other hand, is hot, fast, bright, excited and insubstantial, and is associated with male characteristics and daytime. Anything that is interior, low down, or moving in a downward direction is *yin*. Anything that is exterior, high up, or moving upwards is *yang*.

However, because there is balance in everything, nothing is exclusively *yin* or exclusively *yang* – although it may be predominantly one or the other. There is something of both aspects in everybody and everything. Although a man is predominantly *yang* in his makeup, he has some balancing *yin*. Similarly, a woman has a predominance of *yin*, but she still has a *yang* component.

Western medicine, too, recognises that women have a male component and men a female component. The sex of a foetus is determined at conception – the fusion of an egg with a sperm carrying an X chromosome results in a girl, while fusion with a Y-carrying sperm produces a boy. In their early stages, however, all embryos develop in the same way, regardless of which sex they will ultimately be. The sexual organs develop from the same cells whether the baby is a boy or a girl, and it is at a fairly late stage of intrauterine development that physical differentiation takes place. At birth, all babies are roughly the same shape and, with their clothes on, it is often hard to tell boys from girls. The typical body shape and hair distribution of male and female develop in response to the hormones that are first secreted in large amounts at puberty. Because males can secrete some female hormones and females can secrete some male hormones, it is possible for women to become hairy or for men to develop breast tissue. This can sometimes occur in perfectly normal adolescents while their hormones are, so to speak, sorting themselves out.

You could say that the hairy girl has a temporary excess of *yang*, while the boy whose breasts begin to swell has excessive *yin*. But the terms *yin* and *yang* encompass far more than just sexual characteristics. As components of all animate and inanimate objects, they are in a constant state of flux. According to how you look at something, its '*yin*-ness' and '*yang*-ness' change. For example, when you look at the body as a whole, the outside surface (being exterior) is *yang* and the inner organs (known as the *zang-fu* organs) are *yin*. But if you look only at the trunk, the back is primarily *yang* and the front (or the 'inside' when you bend over) is *yin*. Then again, if you consider the chest and abdomen, the chest (being upper) can be said to be *yang*, and the abdomen (being lower) is *yin*. Thus *yin* and *yang* are not concrete characteristics of an object but are references to that object's relationships to whatever is surrounding it. Here again, the comparison with the concepts of right and left is useful. If you describe your body, you will describe one arm as the left arm and the other as the right arm. However, you could also describe the inside border of your right arm as its left border, or the inside border of your left arm as its right border. So that which is right has an aspect of leftness, and vice versa. Similarly, because we always look at our own bodies from a looking-forward position, our right and left arms remain constant. But if we look at our environment, right and left are variable. Myrtle Crescent may be the first road on the left past the church or the last road on the right before the church, depending on where we are standing when we give the directions.

In all things that are opposite aspects of each other, there has to be balance, since by definition it is the two together that make the whole. You can't have right without left; nor can you recognise light without knowledge of darkness. And the balance that is essential within the body must also be maintained between the body and its environment.

In Western medical terms a fairly simple example of this can be given. Sixty per cent of the body is made up of water, and this water is distributed throughout the body. A certain amount of it is inside the body's cells; some makes up the interstitial fluids that flow around and between the cells, keeping them moist; the rest is in the body's fluids – the blood, lymph, saliva, digestive juices, and other secretions. It is very important that the amount of water in each section remains constant in relation to the others. The body would not be able to function if, when water was drunk, it flowed into a section haphazardly. For example, if excess water entered the bloodstream, the increased blood volume would cause the blood pressure to rise. Similarly, if too much water entered the tissue cells, this would cause oedema (swelling of the tissues). Therefore the body has highly complex mechanisms by which the amount of water taken is apportioned in the correct amounts to the various places where it is needed and so remains balanced.

Anything that has to keep a balance cannot be static or rigid, because it must always be ready to adapt to changes occurring around it. So the balance of *yin* and *yang* must always be fluid. It follows, therefore that any condition that restricts this fluidity will affect the body's ability to maintain its own natural health. In Chinese terms many medical problems are associated with an imbalance of *yin* and *yang*, one or the other being either in excess or deficient. If *yin* becomes excessive, it will overwhelm the *yang* that is trying to balance it. This will result in a disease that has the characteristics of *yin* – coldness, slowness, and lack of activity. But the same type of disease can result if the excess of *yin* is only relative – in other words, if it is due to a deficiency of *yang*. In the same way, an excess of *yang* will overwhelm normal *yin*, producing a disease with *yang* characteristics – heat, excitement and overactivity – which can also be a symptom of a lack of *yin*.

To a physician with Western medical training who is not looking at a patient in terms of *yin* and *yang*, someone with a deficiency of *yang* could appear to have an illness identical to that of another person who is suffering from an excess of *yin*. For example, such symptoms might be exhibited by a patient with myxoedema (thyroid deficiency) who would be treated with a thyroid supplement. However, if a patient with myxoedema were seen by an acupuncturist, she might be diagnosed as having either an excess of *yin* or a deficiency of *yang*. And the acupuncturist would treat the patient with excess *yin* differently from one with deficient *yang*, since he would try to bring back to normal the aspect that was malfunctioning.

The Chinese term for excess or fullness is *shi*, while that for deficiency or 'emptiness' is *xu*. Disease states in which the fundamental problem is one of excess (no matter what the excess) are thus known as *shi* syndromes, while those in which there is a deficiency of any sort are known as *xu* syndromes. A *shi* syndrome may be seen as one in which, although its natural resistance is intact, the body has been invaded and overwhelmed by an outside agent, while a *xu* syndrome is one in which the body's own defences have been lowered to such an extent that it has no resistance. It is clear, therefore, why treatment of the two types of syndrome must differ from each other. In a *xu* syndrome it is necessary to reinforce the body's defences against invasion (for example, deficient *yin* must be stimulated), while in a *shi* syndrome the treatment aims to reduce the excessive factor.

A parallel can be found in Western medical terms. The white blood cells are the body's protection against infection. The production of these cells is dependent on a number of factors, not least on the dietary intake of certain essential nutrients such as zinc, magnesium, vitamin C and vitamin E. If you get an infection, it may be either because your white blood cells are deficient or because the bacteria or viruses are too strong for your body's defences. In the latter case (a *shi* syndrome) antibiotics would be needed to fight the bacteria, but in the former (a *xu* syndrome) it would also be necessary to supplement your diet to reinforce your natural defences. (Many people do this by, for instance, taking large doses of vitamin C to treat a cold.)

A disruption in the balance between *yin* and *yang*, whether it is due to an excess or a deficiency, produces an abnormality in the flow of *qi* in the affected area. When the balance of *yin* and *yang* is restored to normal, the flow of *qi* will also return to normal.

CATEGORIES OF QI

Qi itself can be divided into categories according to the function that it is performing. Having previously said that *qi* is all-pervading and is in a constant state of flux, I realise that this may sound contradictory. However, a parallel with blood may make it clearer. The composition of one person's blood remains the same in terms of the number of red blood cells, white cells and platelets in it, and in terms of the amount of iron in the red cells, no matter where in the body that blood is. However, other things about it will vary according to what its function is at the time. Arterial blood, which has just left the lungs, is carrying oxygen to the body tissues and will be bright red, while venous blood, which is returning to the lungs carrying carbon dioxide to be exhaled, is dark red. The portal vein carries blood containing the broken down products of protein, fats and carbohydrates from the intestines to the liver, while blood entering the kidneys will contain waste products from body cells. But, fundamentally, it is all the same blood; what is venous one minute can become arterial the next simply by passing through the lungs. Similarly, *qi* can be divided into categories. Because it pervades everything, it is seen as being taken in with food and with the air we breathe. Inhaled air contains clean *qi*; exhaled air contains waste *qi*. These, together with the nutrients obtained from food, are known as material *qi*. Nourishing *qi* is derived from the digestion of food by the stomach and spleen and circulates by means of the meridians which carry qi around the body in the same way that the arteries and veins carry the blood. It is these meridians that form the basis for acupuncture therapy. Protective *qi*, which I have mentioned as being the body's natural defence against invasion, is also formed from food and circulates in the superficial tissues of the body and in the skin. Nourishing *qi* is primarily *yin*, whereas protective *qi* is primarily *yang* – again, two aspects of the same thing.

Each organ of the body has its own *qi*, which is known as functional *qi*, and it is this that maintains the normal function of that organ. However, all these different forms of *qi* are both interrelated and interdependent, in exactly the same way that venous blood becomes arterial after it has been through the lungs and arterial blood becomes venous after it has delivered its oxygen to the tissues. The purpose of protective *qi* is to help defend the body from attack by harmful *qi*, which can invade and cause illness. By stimulating and strengthening the level of protective qi, acupuncture can be used as a preventive treatment.

THE MERIDIANS

Acupuncture treatment uses as its medium the meridians through which *qi* flows. The meridians, like the blood vessels, have identical routes on the right and left sides of the body. In the same way that there is a right carotid artery and a left carotid artery, a right renal artery and a left renal artery, and a right femoral vein and a left femoral vein, there are right and left Lung meridians, right and left Kidney meridians and so on. There is, however, a difference. If, for example, there is a malfunction of a vein on the left, in orthodox medicine it is only the left vein that will be treated whereas, in acupuncture, treatment of either the left or the right meridian will affect the other. Some authorities claim that treating only the meridian opposite the one affected will produce an effect in 30 per cent of cases, treating only the affected meridian will produce an effect in 60 per cent, and treating both together will produce an effect in 90 per cent. Other practitioners, more cynical perhaps, say that the reason for this is that if you are inaccurate in locating the acupuncture points, then treatment of both sides gives an increased chance of actually hitting the right spot. Be this as it may, some practitioners always treat patients symmetrically. Aside from this, the fact that treatment of the opposite meridian will affect the disturbed meridian is very valuable when treating a patient in whom pain makes it impossible to treat the affected side. If someone is suffering from shingles, for example, the needles would commonly be put on the side of the body opposite the rash.

There are twelve pairs of meridians. Each half of a pair behaves in exactly the same way as its partner, unless one of them is diseased. It is easier, however, to speak of 'the Lung meridian' rather than of 'the two Lung meridians, left and right'. This therefore, is the terminology that is commonly used and that I will use in this book.

In addition to the twelve major meridians, there are two that are unpaired, known as Du and Ren. They run down the midline of the body, back and front. There are also six other 'extra' meridians that join up points from the major meridians, forming links between them. The meridians are also joined to each other by collaterals; these can be used to carry excess *qi* from one that has too much to another that is deficient.

Each of the twelve major meridians is associated with an organ of the body – thus we have the Lung meridian, the Liver meridian, the Heart meridian and so on. Each meridian receives *qi* from another meridian and passes it on to a third, so that *qi* circulates around the meridians in the same way that blood circulates through the blood vessels. In the latter case a number of factors can affect the amount of blood being carried by a vessel at any one time. For example, after a meal there will be an increased amount of blood in the vessels supplying the stomach and intestines. Or, when the weather is hot, there will be an increased blood supply to the skin so that excess heat can be lost from the body. In contrast, the flow of *qi* through the meridians is controlled by a strict biological clock.

Qi is said to surge in individual meridians at particular times. Each of the twelve major meridians is coupled with one of the others and, while *qi* is surging in one of the couple, it will be at its lowest ebb in the other. So, for example, *qi* is said to be at its maximum in the Liver meridian between 1.00 and 3.00 am, while its opposite number, the Small Intestine meridian, is at its lowest during this period. Between 1.00 and 3.00 pm, however, the position is reversed, with the Small Intestine meridian having its maximum flow of *qi* and the Liver meridian its lowest.

It has been suggested that jet lag may be due to the meridians not yet having adapted to the new time zone in which they have arrived. Going from London to New York, for instance, will find the Liver meridian having its maximum flow at around 8.00 in the evening instead of in the early hours of the morning, which is what it is used to. The symptoms of jet lag will persist until the meridians adapt to the new time zone.

The theory of the circulation of *qi* is of use to the acupuncturist in both the diagnosis and the treatment of his patient. For example, a patient suffering from ulcerative colitis may often be woken by abdominal pain and a need to open her bowels at around 5.00 or 6.00 am. To the acupuncturist, the symptoms plus the timing suggest a disruption of *qi* in the Large Intestine meridian, which has its maximum flow between 5.00 and 7.00 am. It is sometimes helpful, if possible, to treat a meridian during its period of maximum flow, and a patient may therefore be asked to make an appointment for a particular time of day. Obviously, this is more likely to be done with the meridians that have their surges of flow during the day than with those that peak at night, since acupuncturists, like doctors, are unlikely to treat anything other than emergencies at night.

Each meridian is predominantly either *yin* or *yang* (although, of course, each will have aspects of both). In the coupling of meridians, each *yin* meridian is associated with a *yang* meridian, so that when *qi* is at its maximum in a *yin* meridian, it is at its lowest in a *yang* one, and vice versa. The circulation of *qi* around the meridians entails it passing through two *yin* meridians, followed by two *yang* meridians, then two *yin* meridians, and so on. Each *yin* meridian is associated with a so-called solid, or *zang*, organ, while *yang* meridians are associated with hollow, or *fu*, organs. This relates back to the association of *yin* with solidity and *yang* with lack of substance.

When looked at anatomically, not all the 'solid' organs are truly solid, so it might be more appropriate to refer to them by the Chinese terms, *zang* and *fu*. The *zang* organs are the heart, the liver, the spleen, the lung, the kidney and the pericardium. (The pericardium is the fibrous sac that surrounds the heart and assists its contraction. In some Western books on acupuncture it is referred to as the heart constrictor.) The *fu* organs are the small intestine, the large intestine, the stomach, the gallbladder, the urinary bladder and the *sanjiao*. The last of these is a Chinese concept and not an organ in its own right in Western terms. The word *sanjiao* may be translated as 'three warmers' or 'triple warmer' and refers to the chest (the upper *jiao*), the upper abdomen (middle *jiao*) and the lower abdomen (lower *jiao*) which are related to each other by their function of warming the organs contained within them.

The routes taken by the meridians are also related to their *yin* or *yang* qualities – the *yin* meridians of the arms and legs run down their inner aspects, while the *yang* meridians run down the outside.

Each meridian is intimately related to the organ from which it gets is name. So the Lung meridian extends into the lung, the Liver meridian into the liver, the Large Intestine meridian into the large bowel, and so on. The organs themselves can be affected by treatment of the corresponding meridian, and disorders of a particular meridian may manifest as symptoms associated with its organ. The diagrams on the following pages illustrate the part of the meridian that is used in treatment – in other words, the part that runs near the surface of the body and along which the acupuncture points lie. But they tell only half the story because these surface meridians extend into internal meridians, which are the links between the acupuncture points and the internal organs.

The Lung meridian, which is *yin*, runs superficially from just below the collar bone, down the inside of the arm and into the thumb, where it ends next to the nail. This is shown in figure 1. The Lung meridian is usually put first in any list of the meridians, since it is seen as being the starting point in the cycle of *qi*. It has a surge of energy between 3.00 and 5.00 am, at which time its coupled meridian – that of the Urinary Bladder – is at its lowest.

There are eleven acupuncture points lying along the course of the meridian and these are referred to either by their Chinese names or else as Lung 1, Lung 2 (often abbreviated to Lu 1, Lu 2) and so on.

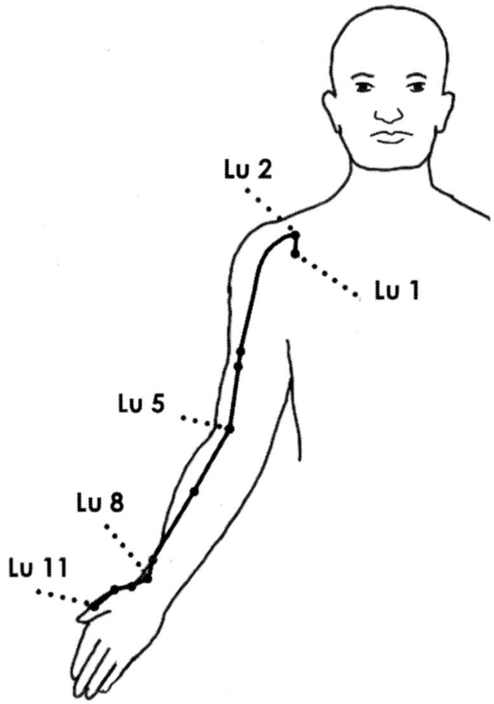

Figure 1 - Lung meridian

Interruption of the flow of *qi* in the Lung meridian and consequent disruption of its function may cause symptoms such as cough, asthma, or tightness in the chest (all associated with the internal course of the meridian and its link with the lungs), or symptoms in the arms along the course of the superficial part of the meridian. When disruption affects a single meridian, either wholly or predominantly, the symptoms produced by an excess or a deficiency of *qi* will be related to the function and course of that meridian and may be diagnostic. (More will be said about excess and deficiency syndromes in the next chapter.)

An excess in the Lung meridian may produce a heavy feeling in the chest, shortness of breath, a severe cough with copious sputum, a dry and sore throat, a nasal discharge, redness of the bridge of the nose, and pain in the shoulder and arm. A deficiency may result in sneezing, a dry cough, dry skin, faintness, weight loss, shallow breathing, sensitivity to cold, and redness of the chin.

Figure 2 shows the Large Intestine meridian, which is the first of the two *yang* meridians that come immediately after the Lung meridian in the daily cycle of *qi*. It surges between 5.00 and 7.00 am when the Kidney meridian, with which it is coupled, is at its lowest.

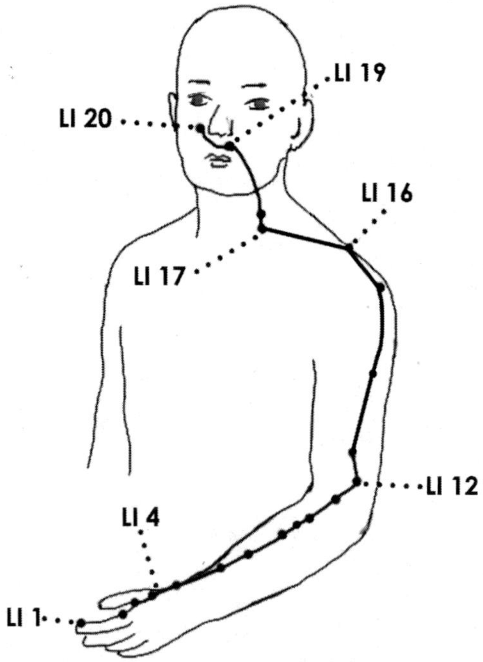

Figure 2 - Large Intestine meridian

Because the Large Intestine meridian receives *qi* directly from the Lung meridian, it begins very close to the end of the latter, its first point being next to the nail of the index finger.

It is a *yang* meridian, so its course up the arm is along the outer aspect. Since it terminates very close to the nose, disruption of this meridian may be associated with nosebleeds. In addition, because it passes across the lower part of the face, it may be implicated in toothache. Sore throat and pain in the shoulder or arm are associated with the position of the rest of its superficial course. And because of its internal links with the large intestine itself, abdominal pain and diarrhoea may also be symptoms of disruption of this meridian.

An excess in the meridian is likely to cause pain along its course, stiffness of the shoulder, dizziness, abdominal distension, and constipation, while a deficiency may result in diarrhoea, shivering, and a dry mouth.

The Large Intestine meridian has twenty points along its superficial course, which are listed as LI 1, LI 2 and so on up to LI 20. In some books it is called the Colon meridian (colon being another name for the major part of the large intestine) in which case it is abbreviated to Co 1, Co 2 and so on.

From the Large Intestine meridian, *qi* runs down the *yang* Stomach meridian, which is shown in figures 3a and 3b. Here again, the fact that it is a *yang* meridian is reflected in its course which, when it runs down the leg, does so along the outer aspect. The Stomach meridian has its surge of *qi* between 7.00 and 9.00 am, when the Pericardium meridian is at its lowest.

Disruption of the flow of *qi* in the Stomach meridian may produce symptoms associated with any part of its superficial course, such as nosebleed, sore throat, or chest pain. Symptoms related to the stomach itself, such as indigestion or upper abdominal pain, may also occur.

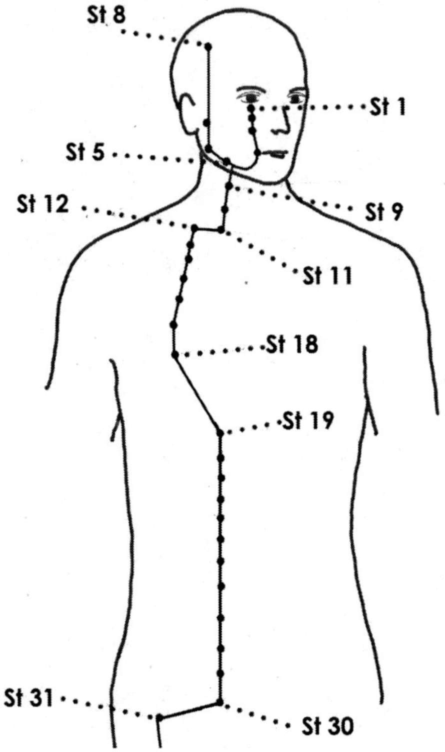

Figure 3a - Stomach meridian, upper section

An excess in the meridian may cause increased appetite, constipation, thirst, bad breath, swelling and pain in the mouth, cramps in the legs, and fever. A deficiency may produce distension of the abdomen, diarrhoea, vomiting, loss of appetite, and weakness in the legs. Forty five points lie along the Stomach meridian, abbreviated to St 1, up to St 45.

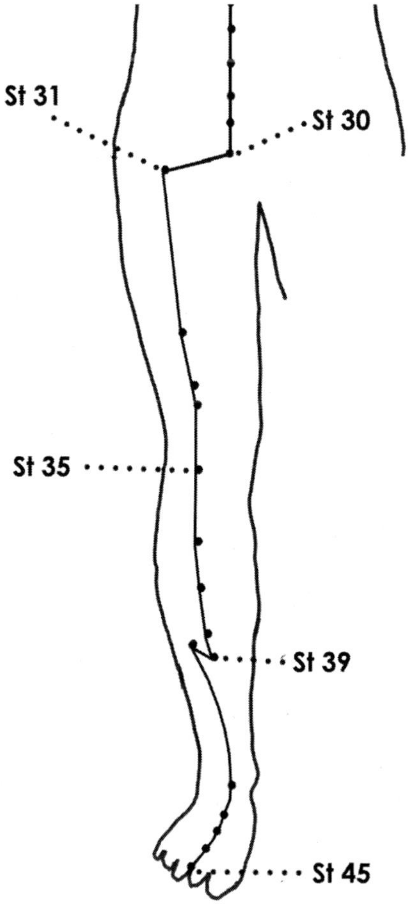

Figure 3b - Stomach meridian, lower section

The *yin* Spleen meridian continues the course of *qi*, travelling from the big toe up the leg (along the inside, since it is a *yin* meridian) and over the abdomen to end a little way below the armpit. Its course is shown in figures 4a and 4b.

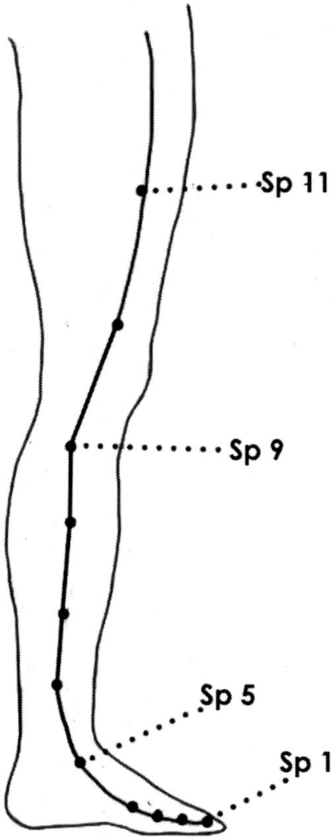

Figure 4a - Spleen meridian, lower section

Interference with its function may cause vomiting, upper abdominal pain, jaundice, or diarrhoea, all of which are related to its internal course and its path across the abdomen; or it may produce symptoms further down its course, such as painful or swollen knees. An excess affecting this meridian is likely to cause congestion in the chest, with a productive cough, constipation, fatigue, and an irregular appetite.

A deficiency may cause diarrhoea and vomiting, flatulence, water retention, sleepiness, heaviness of the legs, and a poor memory. The Spleen meridian has twenty points, Sp 1 to Sp 20, and its surge of *qi* comes between 9.00 and 11.00 am, the Sanjiao meridian having the lowest flow at this time.

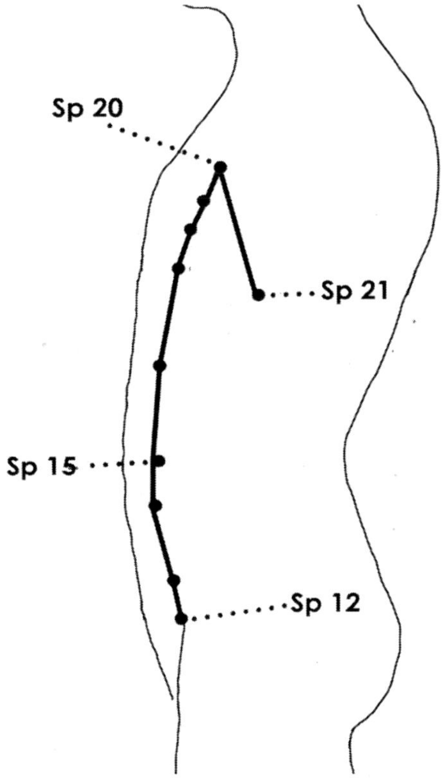

Figure 4b - Spleen meridian, upper section

From the end of the Spleen meridian, *qi* is taken up by the *yin* Heart meridian which runs from the armpit down the inside of the arm and into the little finger, as shown in figure 5. The Heart meridian is one of the two shortest meridians (the Pericardium meridian being the other), with only nine points along its course, H 1 to H 9. Disruption of this meridian can cause symptoms that tie in well with the Western concept of heart disease, such as chest pain, palpitations, and pain in the arms, but because the heart in Chinese medicine is said to be the seat of the mind or spirit, it can also produce symptoms such as insomnia. An excess may be associated with a feeling of heaviness in the chest and a fever, while a deficiency may cause cold sweats, restlessness, palpitations and a poor memory. The *qi* in the Heart meridian (which is coupled with the Gall Bladder meridian) surges between 11.00 am and 1.00 pm.

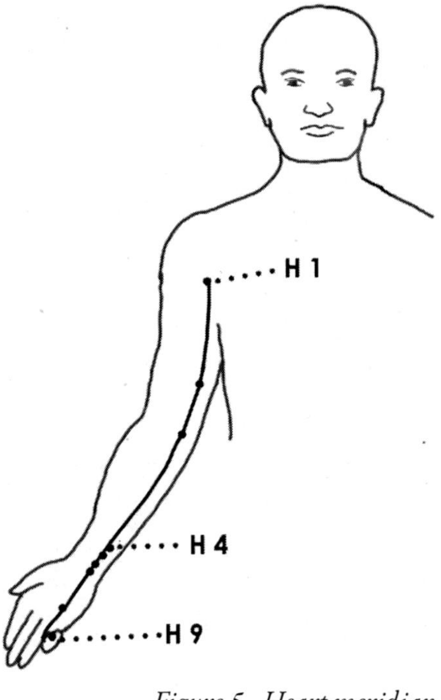

Figure 5 - Heart meridian

Figure 6 shows how, from the little finger, it flows out again via the *yang* Small Intestine meridian up the outer (*yang*) aspect of the arm to just in front of the ear. Disruption of the Small Intestine meridian can produce deafness, sore throat, or pain in the shoulder and arm, all of which are related to its course, or abdominal pain which is related to its inner links with the small bowel. Cold sores may be associated with an excess in this meridian, as may pain in the neck and shoulder.

Ringing in the ears and a tender abdomen may be signs of a deficiency. Nineteen points lie along its course, shown as SI 1 to SI 19. *Qi* in the Small Intestine meridian surges between 1.00 and 3.00 pm, when the flow in the Liver meridian is at its lowest.

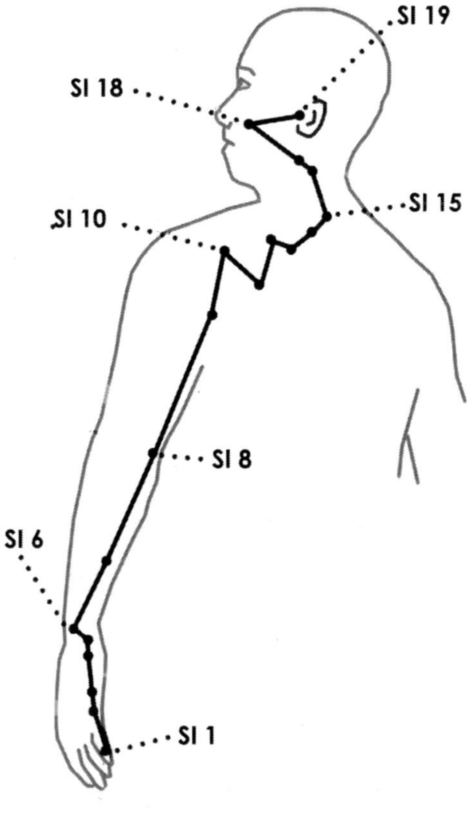

Figure 6 - Small Intestine meridian

Following on from the Small Intestine meridian, the *yang* Urinary Bladder meridian (sometimes referred to just as the Bladder meridian) carries *qi* from the area between the eye and the nose up across the head, down through the neck, and along the side of the spine to the leg, where it travels down the back of the leg and into the foot to end in the little toe. Its route is shown in figures 7a, 7b, 7c and 7d. As you can see, the Urinary Bladder meridian also has an extra branch, which runs down the length of the spine parallel to the first channel.

Urinary problems are, naturally, associated with malfunction of this meridian. Pain anywhere along the length of the spine may also be a result of disruption of the flow of *qi* in the Urinary Bladder meridian.

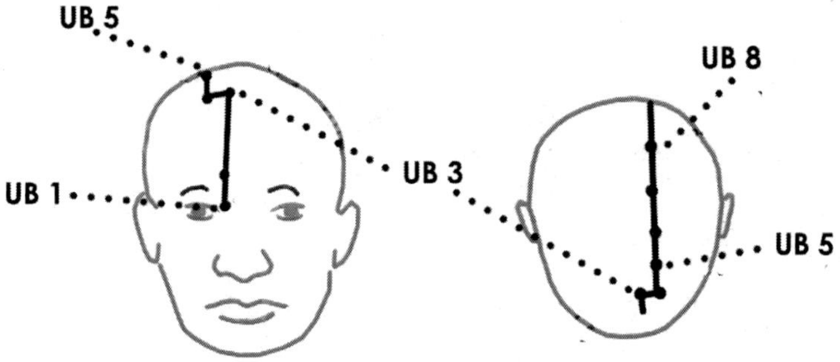

Figure 7a - Urinary Bladder meridian, on the head

Because the channel starts its external course just between the nose and the eye, injury to it may be responsible for nasal congestion, nosebleeds, headaches, watering eyes, and other eye problems. Frequent urination or bed-wetting may occur as a result of a deficiency in the meridian.

I mentioned in connection with its paired meridian, that of the Lung, that the Urinary Bladder meridian is at its lowest ebb of energy between 3.00 and 5.00 am. This, of course, is a period of the night that is commonly associated with bed-wetting in children and it is also the time at which many older people find it necessary to get up in order to empty their bladders.

The surge of energy in the Urinary Bladder meridian comes at the opposite end of the day, between 3.00 and 5.00 in the afternoon. It is the longest of the meridians, mainly due to its parallel tracks down the back.

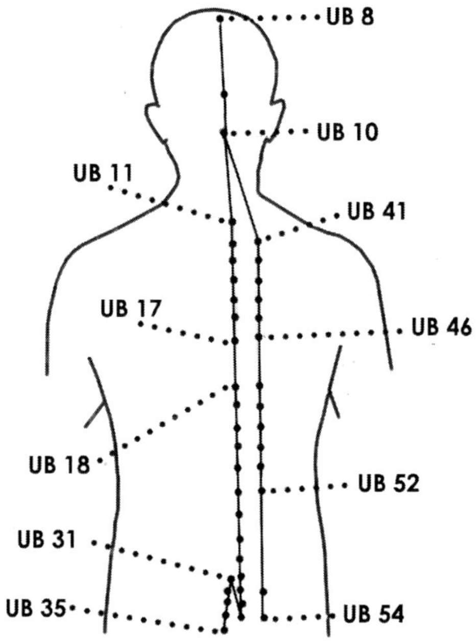

Figure 7b - Urinary Bladder meridian - upper section

There are sixty seven points, commonly abbreviated to UB 1 to UB 67 (or Bl 1 to Bl 67 if it is being referred to simply as the Bladder meridian). However, the numbering of points along this meridian is not consistent in all books. Some authorities (mainly Chinese) number the points starting at the eye and going down to the base of the spine (UB 1 to UB 35), then from below the buttock to the knee (UB 36 to UB 40), followed by the parallel course in the back (UB 41 to UB 54) and, finally, the section below the knee to the end of the meridian (UB 55 to UB 67). This is the system shown in figures 7a-7d. The other system of numbering, which seems to be favoured in America, takes the sections in a different order so that, after the first section (which remains the same), the parallel course in the back becomes UB 36 to UB 49 and the final section goes from below the buttock to the foot and is numbered UB 50 to UB 67.

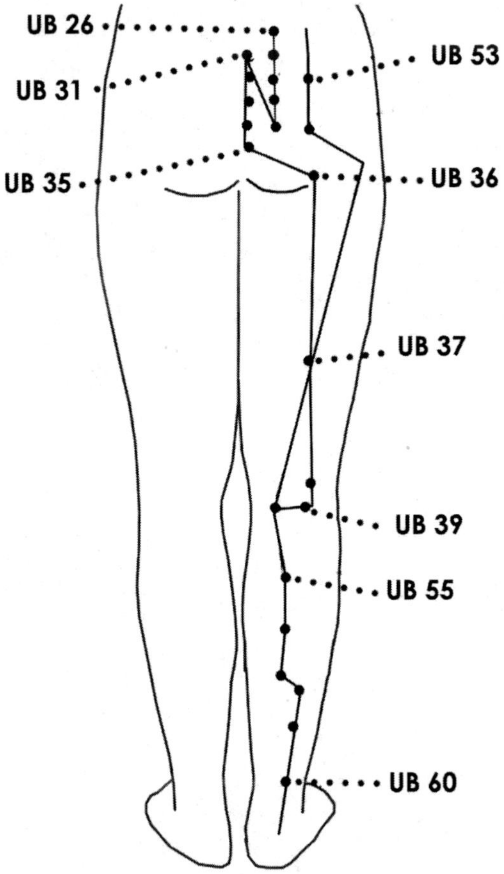

Figure 7c - Urinary Bladder meridian, lower section

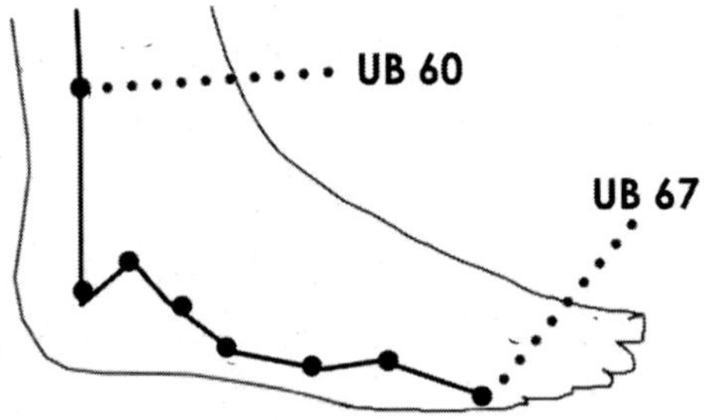

Figure 7d - Urinary Bladder meridian, on the foot

Next in the cycle is the *yin* Kidney meridian, which is shown in figures 8a and 8b. It begins, as you might guess, near the end of the Urinary Bladder meridian, in the foot. Beginning on the sole, it runs up the leg (along the inside, since it is a *yin* channel) and then up the abdomen, near the midline, to finish just below the inner aspect of the collarbone. It has its surge of energy between 5.00 and 7.00 pm, and the twenty seven points that lie along its course are abbreviated to K 1 to K 27.

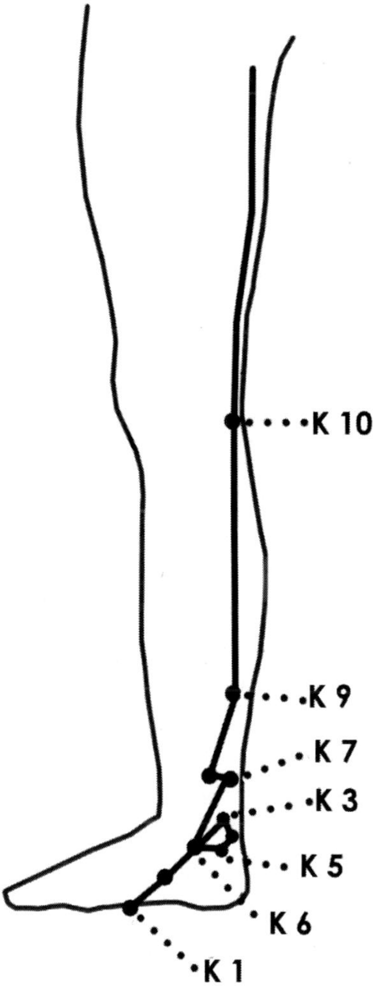

Figure 8a - Kidney meridian, lower section

Abnormalities of the Kidney meridian, like those of the Urinary Bladder meridian, may be associated urinary problems. However, in addition, the Kidney meridian regulates sexual function, so disruption of its flow of *qi* may cause menstrual problems in women or impotence in men. Its course across the chest means that asthma, coughing of blood, and sore throat may all be associated with problems in the this meridian, and its course down the leg may produce local pain as a symptom of malfunction.

An excess in the meridian may cause the patient to become hyperactive, while a deficiency can produce a loss of sex drive and a general timidity. Both excess and deficiency can be associated with ringing in the ears (more will be said about the kidney's link with the ears later on).

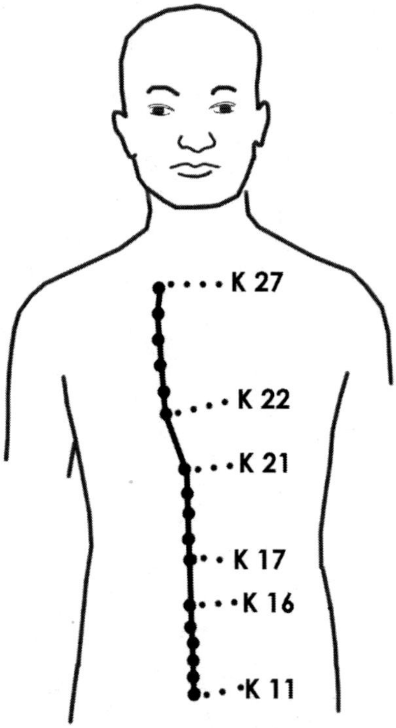

Figure 8b - Kidney meridian, upper section

Following on from the Kidney meridian is the *yin* Pericardium meridian. Like the Heart meridian, with which it is closely associated, it has only nine points, listed as P 1 to P 9 (or, in some books, as HC 1 to HC 9, where HC stands for Heart Constrictor).

The course of the Pericardium meridian runs more or less parallel to that of the Heart meridian, as can be seen in figure 9. Since the pericardium surrounds the heart, its meridian is associated with heart problems, including chest pain, palpitations, and shortness of breath. Malfunction of the Pericardium meridian can also produce anxiety and mental disturbance (because the heart is the seat of the mind).

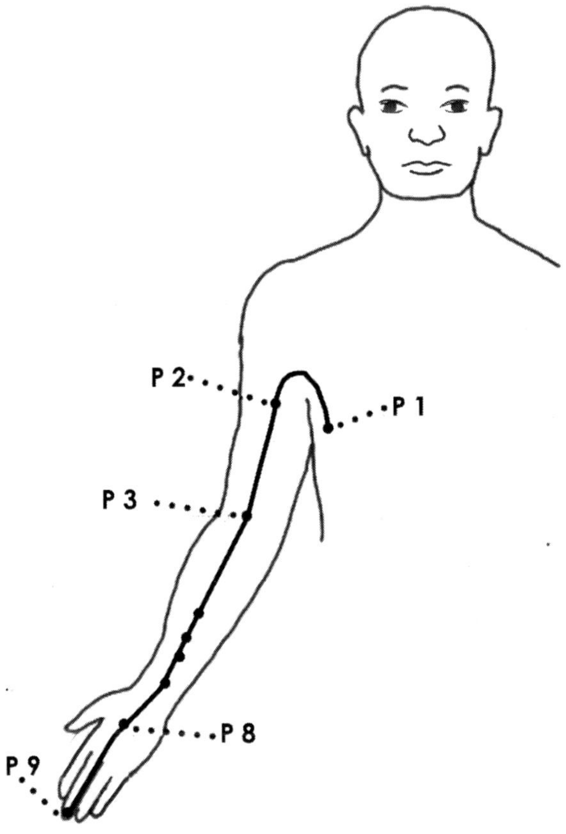

Figure 9 - Pericardium meridian

Headache, abdominal pain, and fever may be associated with an excess affecting the Pericardium meridian, while a deficiency can cause palpitations, shortness of breath, indigestion, and diarrhoea. Restless sleep may result from either an excess or a deficiency. *Qi* surges through the Pericardium meridian between 7.00 and 9.00 pm.

The *yang* Sanjiao meridian, shown in figure 10, follows on from the Pericardium meridian and carries *qi* from the ring finger up the arm (the outer aspect, since it is a *yang* meridian) into the shoulder, up the side of the neck, and around the ear to finish next to the outer end of the eyebrow. Sanjiao is often translated as Triple Heater, Triple Burner or Triple Energiser, so its twenty three points can be shown with the abbreviation SJ (as in this book), TH, TB or TE.

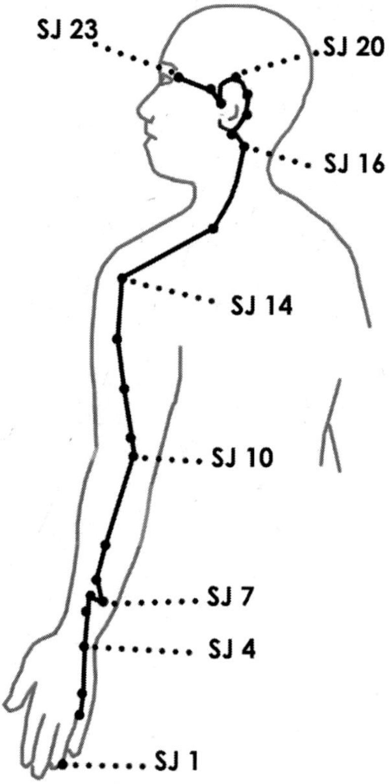

Figure 10 - Sanjiao meridian

Disruption of the Sanjiao meridian can cause problems associated with any of the three cavities. For example, abdominal pain or distension may relate to the middle cavity, or jiao, and pain on passing urine to the lower jiao. But symptoms may also be related simply to the course of the meridian. These include ringing in the ears, sore throat, and pain in the shoulders or arms. Such pain may relate to an excess in the meridian, as may sore throat, hearing difficulties, constipation, and retention of urine. A deficiency may be associated with nervousness and restlessness, diarrhoea, incontinence, or water retention.

The *yang* Gall Bladder meridian, whose energy surges between 11.00 pm and 1.00 am, follows on from the Sanjiao meridian. Its long and somewhat convoluted route is shown in figures 11a and 11b. Here again, as a *yang* meridian, it runs down the outside of the leg.

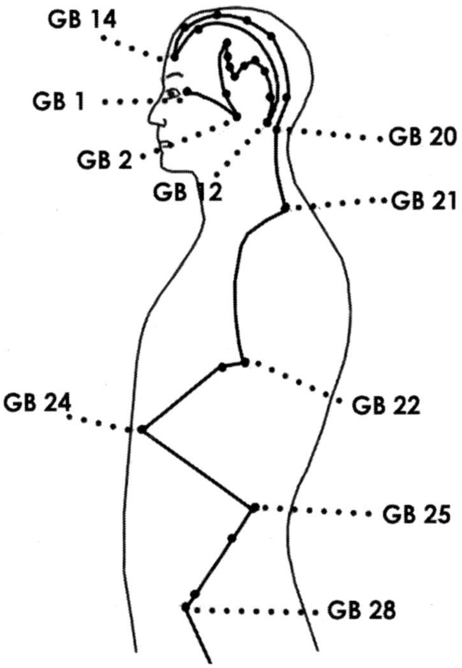

Figure 11a - Gall Bladder meridian, upper section

Disruption of the flow of *qi* may cause symptoms related to any part of its superficial course, such as headache, blurring of vision, or pain affecting the chest, upper abdomen, or legs. An excess in the meridian may produce an increased appetite, abdominal pain, or jaundice, while deficiency may be responsible for dizziness, anxiety, and insomnia. Forty four points, GB 1 to GB 44, lie along its course.

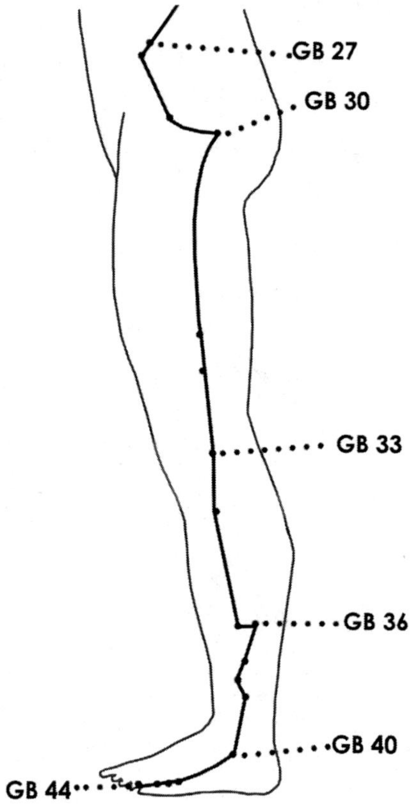

Figure 11b - Gall Bladder meridian, lower section

The Liver meridian is a *yin* meridian which runs, as you can see in figures 12a and 12b, from the big toe up the inside of the leg to the trunk, where it ends just below the nipple. This meridian is at its highest point of energy between 1.00 and 3.00 in the morning. Disruption of its function may be associated with pain anywhere along its superficial course, but particularly in the lower abdomen, and on passing water. Its course passes through the groin, and therefore hernias may be associated with its malfunction. So, too, may a feeling of tightness in the lower part of the chest and hiccups (which are due to spasmodic contractions of the diaphragm – the large sheet of muscle attached to the lower border of the ribs that separates the abdomen from the chest).

The liver itself is said to have specific functions, which I will describe in the next chapter. These are not the same functions as those accorded to it in Western medicine, and they may be disrupted by malfunction of the Liver meridian, producing symptoms such as headache and mental disturbance.

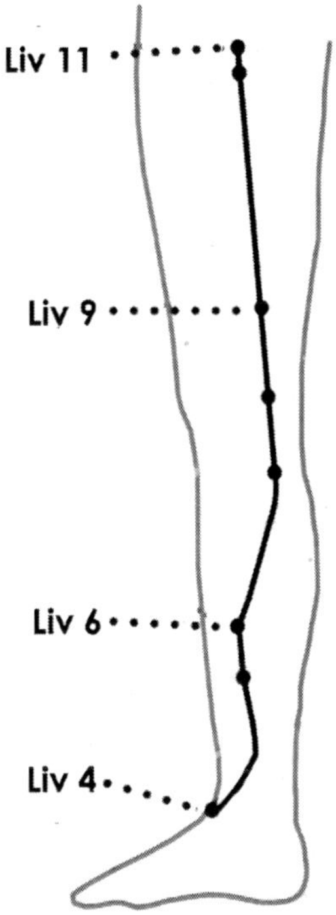

Figure 12a - Liver meridian, lower section

An excess in the meridian may be associated with an unstable temperament, hyperactivity, and abdominal pain, while a deficiency may cause dizziness, poor eyesight, and dry skin. The Liver meridian has fourteen points, usually abbreviated Liv 1 to Liv 14 but shown as Li 1 to Li 14 in some books.

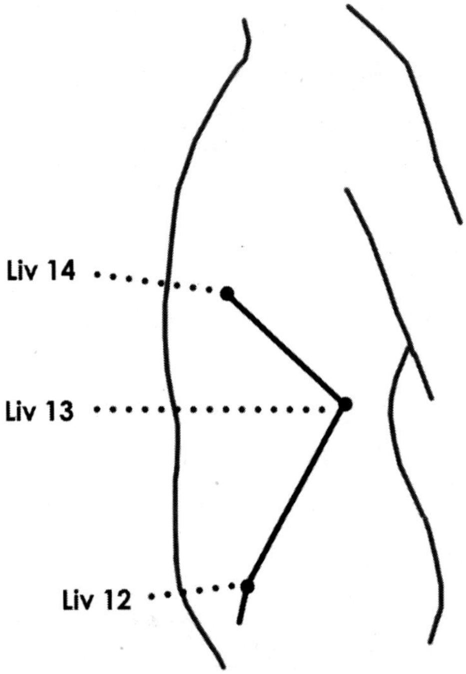

Figure 12b - Liver meridian, upper section

From the Liver meridian, the circulation of *qi* is completed by the Lung meridian, which picks it up again under the collarbone.

There are also two midline meridians, Du and Ren, whose courses are shown in figures 13a, 13b and 14.

The Du meridian (sometimes called the Governing Vessel) has twenty eight points, shown either as Du 1 to Du 28 or as GV 1 to GV 28. It runs up the midline of the body from the base of the spine over the head to the centre of the top lip. It forms a circle with the Ren meridian, also known as the Vessel of Conception.

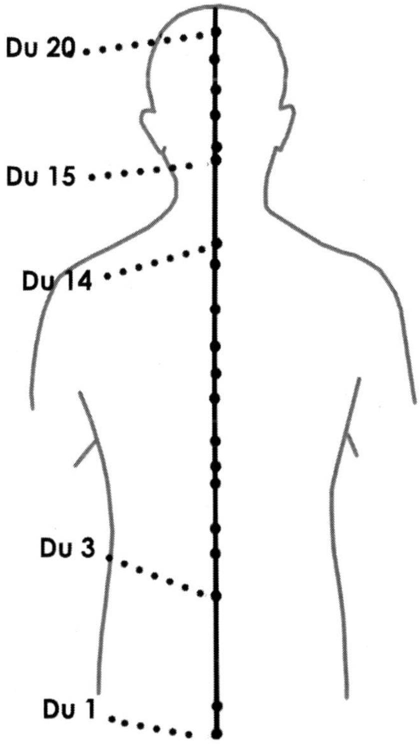

Figure 13a - Du meridian, posterior

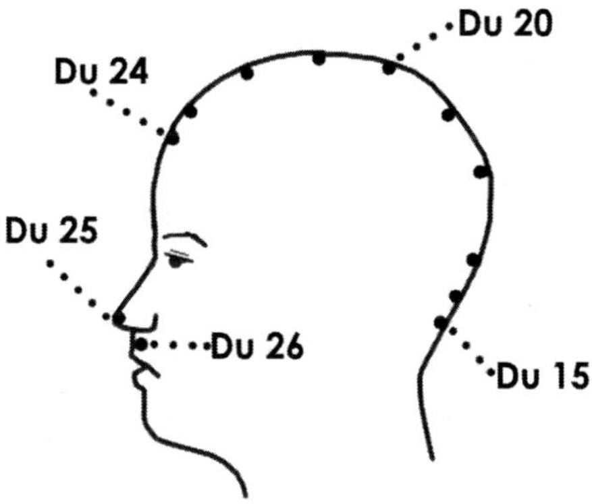

Figure 13b - Du meridian, on the head

The Ren meridian has twenty four points (Ren 1 to Ren 24 or VC 1 to VC 24) and runs from the centre of the perineum (the area between the legs, in front of the anus) up the midline of the abdomen and chest, to finish just below the centre of the lower lip. The Du meridian is *yang* since it runs down the back, or outside, of the body, while the Ren meridian, running down the front, or inside, is *yin*. Disruption of the Du meridian may be associated with back pain and headache.

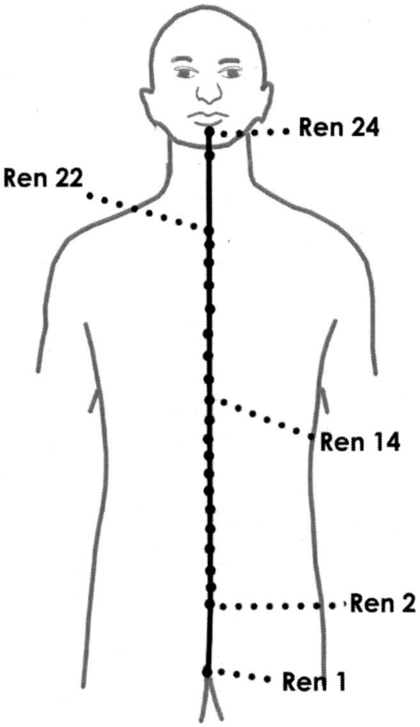

Figure 14 - Ren meridian

Abnormalities in the Ren meridian are associated with menstrual problems, vaginal discharge, retention of urine, and abdominal pain.

There are also extra meridians that link points from the other main meridians. For example, the Yangwei meridian (a *yang* meridian, naturally) runs through points on the *yang* Urinary Bladder, Gall Bladder, Small Intestine, Sanjiao, Stomach and Du meridians, while the Yingwei meridian (a *yin* meridian) joins points on the *yin* Kidney, Spleen, Liver and Ren meridians.

Finally, there are also twenty extra points that are not connected with any specific meridian. Since *qi* must, by its nature, circulate through the entire body, an acupuncture point does not necessarily have to be on a meridian, in the same way that you do not have to cut through a vein or artery in order to bleed.

There are 309 points on the paired meridians – counted only from one side of the body since these meridians are mirror images of each other and Liv 1, for example, will be Liv 1 whether it is on the right or the left side. So the total number of individually named acupuncture points from the twelve meridians, the two Du and Ren meridians, and the extra points is 381 – 309 plus 28 plus 24 plus 20. It is interesting to note that the Yellow Emperor's Classic refers to 365 points, demonstrating that very little has changed in the basic theory of acupuncture in two thousand years.

3

THE FIVE ELEMENTS

Each of the twelve major meridians is related to one of the elements recognised in classical Chinese philosophy – Earth, Wood, Water, Metal and Fire. These elements are understood to be intimately associated with all things, including the human body. Fire is associated with four meridians, while the other elements are associated with two meridians each. In some cases, the reasoning behind the association is obvious (for example, the Urinary Bladder and Kidney meridians are linked to Water). In others, it is understandable (such as the linkage of the Heart meridian with Fire). In yet others, such as the association of the Gall Bladder meridian with Wood, we have to take it on trust. In addition to the overall association with one specific element, each meridian has five acupuncture points that are related to each of the five elements.

One of the fundamentals of holistic theory is that no one part of the body can be disrupted in any way, no matter how small, without it having an effect on other parts. Figure 15 shows how the meridians and their associated elements are related to each other according to the Law of the Five Elements. Disruption of the flow of *qi* in one meridian is likely, directly or indirectly, to affect others. This means that the meridian to which the patient's symptoms appear to be related is not necessarily the meridian that needs treating. The underlying cause may be in another meridian, whose disruption has caused abnormalities to occur in the symptom-producing meridian.

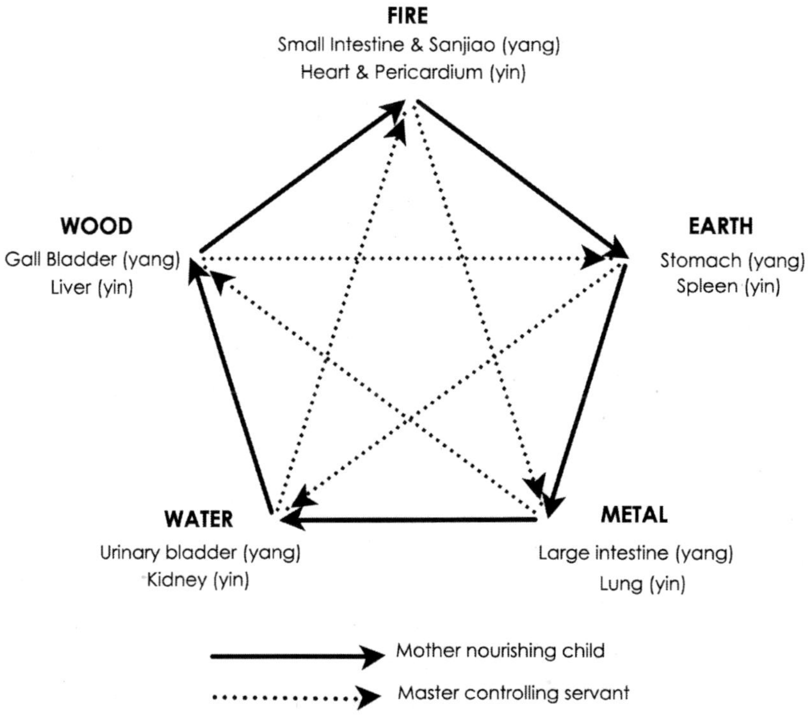

Figure 15 - The Five Elements

The rules that govern the effects of elements on each other, and therefore of meridians on each other, are known as the mother-child rule and the servant-master rule. It is said that, in the same way that a mother gives birth to a child and nourishes him, so elements promote and nourish other elements. Wood is said to promote Fire because it is combustible; a log fire that is deprived of wood to burn will go out. Fire, in turn, promotes Earth by creating ashes. Even nowadays, certain forms of ash are used as fertilisers to nourish the earth. Earth promotes Metal because metal is dug out of the earth and so is engendered by it. Metal promotes Water – with a stretch of the imagination – by melting. And Water promotes Wood by nourishing the tree, because a tree that is deprived of water will die.

By analogy, then, when a meridian associated with Wood (the Liver or the Gall

Bladder meridian) is functioning normally, it will promote normal flow of *qi* and normal function in the Fire meridians (Heart, Pericardium, Small Intestine, and Sanjiao). In turn the normal function of the Fire meridians promotes flow in the Earth meridians (Spleen and Stomach) which, in the same way, nourish the Metal meridians (Lung and Large Intestine). These promote the function of the Water meridians (Urinary Bladder and Kidney) which complete the circle by nourishing the Wood meridians.

It follows that disruption to the flow of *qi* in one meridian can disrupt flow in the meridian that it normally nourishes. If the disruption is allowed to continue untreated, it may go a step further, affecting the meridian that is nourished by the second meridian involved. In this way the condition can spread to involve the entire body and meridian system.

The servant-master rule produces a different cycle of events. It is said that, just as a master gives orders to his servant and controls his actions, so elements affect others by maintaining control over them. It is this control by the master, as much as the nourishment obtained from the mother, that enables the element in question to function normally. Wood is said to control Earth, since trees grow on it and over it. Earth, in turn controls Water by damming it and so forcing it to flow in certain directions. Water controls Fire, naturally enough, by extinguishing it, and Fire controls Metal by melting it. Metal controls Wood by being made into tools that can cut it and fashion it into other things, and this completes the circle. So the Wood meridians (Liver and Gall Bladder) exert control over the Earth meridians (Spleen and Stomach). These two then control the Water meridians (Urinary Bladder and Kidney), which control the Fire meridians (Small Intestine, Sanjiao, Heart and Pericardium). The Fire meridians control the Metal meridians (Lung and Large Intestine), and the latter control the Wood meridians. A malfunction in a meridian may be produced by a malfunction in which the master meridian exerts either inadequate or excessive control over its servant. In the latter case, the *qi* of the servant meridian may be reduced or – if the servant 'rebels' against the increased control – may be excessive.

According to the Law of the Five Elements, each meridian has four connections. It is nourished by one meridian and controlled by another. It nourishes a third and controls a fourth. So each element is connected with every other element, as figure 15 shows, either as a mother, a child, a master or a servant. In this respect, the *yin* meridians primarily affect and are affected by the other *yin* meridians, and the *yang* meridians primarily affect and are affected by the other *yang* meridians.

It may be helpful here to look at one meridian and see how it can be affected by other meridians according to the mother-child and the servant-master rules. If we take as our example the Heart meridian – a *yin* Fire meridian – we will see that it is nourished by its mother, the Liver meridian (the *yin* Wood meridian) and in turn nourishes its child, the Spleen meridian (the *yin* Earth meridian). It is controlled by its master, the Kidney meridian (the *yin* Water meridian) and exerts control over its servant, the Lung meridian (the *yin* Metal meridian).

It follows from this that a malfunction of the Heart meridian may be intimately related to a malfunction of the Liver, Spleen, Kidney or Lung meridians. If the disorder originated in one of the other meridians, then treatment of the Heart meridian alone will not resolve the problem. The whole system must be balanced before the body can become healthy again.

I have heard a Western medical practitioner say that he thought acupuncture must be an easy therapy to master as "you just have to learn what each point does and then stick in your needles". But what I have just said about the Law of the Five Elements should make it clear that this is not the case. Acupuncture is not about diseases but about energy flow. And therefore it is not a question of learning that "this point cures headache and that one will stop vomiting". Each point has a specific function, sure enough, but this function has to do with moving energies around. And so, before practitioners can use the points correctly, they must learn not only what each point does but also how to make a diagnosis in terms of what has gone wrong with the energy flow. Admittedly, there are some points with specific actions, such as the control of vomiting, but to use points only for this type of action without any knowledge of the theory of the flow of *qi* is to use acupuncture at a fairly primitive level. The difference, perhaps, is similar to that between someone with a first aid certificate and a surgeon. The former may certainly be useful in an emergency, but if he tried to ape the surgeon's work, it is likely that he would end up doing more harm than good. To learn the basic theory of acupuncture in order to use it fully, correctly, and in a truly holistic way takes at least three years. The skill of the acupuncturist lies in diagnosing where the imbalance of *qi* lies, and in order to do this she has to know all the laws that govern both the meridians and the *qi* flowing in them. I will say more about diagnosis in the next chapter.

Let us return now to the Heart meridian which, as we have seen, is closely related though the Law of the Five Elements to the Liver, Spleen, Kidney and Lung meridians. According to this law, a deficiency of *qi* in its mother Liver meridian could cause the Heart meridian to become undernourished so that it, too, develops a deficiency. Similarly, an excess of *qi* in the Liver meridian could spill over and cause *qi* in the Heart meridian to become excessive. A deficiency originating in the Heart meridian itself would deprive its child, the Spleen meridian. Any condition in which the symptoms appear to be related to one meridian but are in fact due to a deficiency in the mother meridian is known as the screaming child syndrome – and the child will go on screaming until it is nourished.

A deficiency in the Heart meridian could also track backwards in the cycle and produce a deficiency in the Liver meridian by 'sucking it dry'. An excess of *qi* can also be transmitted either way, from mother to child or from child to mother. If a deficiency or an excess is found in the Liver, Heart and Spleen meridians, this may well have originated from a primary disorder of the Heart meridian. In such a case, treatment of the Heart meridian alone may resolve the problem.

The liver itself, as distinct from its meridian, is said by traditional Chinese physicians to store blood and control the volume of the circulating blood. But the function of the liver is dependent on the normality of its related meridian. If there is a deficiency of *qi* in the Liver meridian, not only *qi* but also blood may be deficient. This would have an effect on its child, the Heart meridian, and on its child's related organ, the heart.

Western medicine also recognises a link between the liver and the heart, although it is not expressed in the same terms as in traditional Chinese medicine. The liver is the storehouse for various vitamins and minerals, including iron and vitamin B12, which are essential for normal blood formation. A deficiency in the liver in Western terms (that is, a depletion of its nutritional stores) may have a serious effect on the blood, causing anaemia. If severe enough, this may put stress on the heart and affect its action.

Another intimate relationship acknowledged by Western medicine is between the spleen and the heart – in Chinese terms, the child and its mother. Red blood cells, which are responsible for carrying oxygen in the blood, have a life span of about 120 days. As cells reach this age, they are broken down by the spleen and the iron that is released from them is reused by the bone marrow to produce new red blood cells. There are some forms of anaemia – known as haemolytic anaemias – in which excessive quantities of red blood cells, young as well as old, are broken down. This may put the heart under strain. Indeed, a sudden and overwhelming haemolytic crisis may precipitate heart failure. Although Chinese medicine does not describe the physiological function of the spleen in breaking down old red blood cells, it says that the spleen is the organ responsible for controlling the blood inside the blood vessels and preventing it from leaking out.

As we have seen, good health entails a normal balance between the *qi* of all the meridians. If a meridian fails, it may lose its control over its servant meridian. In this way a failing Kidney meridian can lose control over its servant, the Heart meridian, or a failing Heart meridian (in the role of the master) can lose control over the Lung meridian. A similar sort of relationship whereby one system is controlled by another is understood in Western medicine. For example, a hormone is produced by the pituitary gland that stimulates the thyroid gland to produce hormones of its own. High levels of circulating thyroid hormones should cause the pituitary to switch off its hormone secretion, whereas low levels should stimulate it – but this biofeedback mechanism can break down. A patient with an overactive or underactive thyroid gland may therefore have a problem either in the gland itself or in the pituitary which has, so to speak, lost control.

The servant-master relationship is therefore one in which overactivity or underactivity of a meridian or its related organ may be associated with a loss of control or an excess of control by the master meridian. The Kidney meridian controls the Heart meridian, and the Heart meridian controls the Lung meridian. These three organs, the kidney, heart and lung, are also recognised by Western physicians as being intimately related to each other. The function of the kidneys is to maintain a balance of water and of minerals within the body. They also eliminate waste products, drugs and other toxins from the body by filtering these, together with water and minerals, out of the blood and then returning to the clean blood exactly the right amounts of water and minerals to keep the body in balance. The waste matter, rejected matter, and excess water are excreted as urine. If the kidneys fail to function normally, there is a build-up of toxins in the body, as well as retention of water and excessive minerals. The result is a rise in blood pressure. This affects the heart (whose meridian, according to Chinese theory, is controlled by that of the kidney). A continually raised blood pressure may finally result in heart failure, and this, in turn, causes fluid to accumulate in the lungs. In the West, this would be called pulmonary oedema but, looked at through an acupuncturist's eyes, it might be seen as a case of the heart failing to control the lungs. As we shall see in the next chapter, the lung is one of the organs said by the Chinese to be responsible for the normal distribution of water around the body.

These relationships have been expressed here in rather simplistic terms. In fact, in both Western and Chinese medicine, the picture is somewhat more complicated. However, it does help to demonstrate how, in both systems, the functions of these organs are interrelated.

The meridians that relate to each other as mother-child and servant-master are linked by specific points, the needling of which can open a channel between the two in order to allow *qi* to flow from one to the other and so return to a state of equilibrium. Various points are available on each meridian by which transfer of *qi* can be effected, and every meridian has a point relating to each of the elements – Earth, Water, Fire, Metal and Wood. These points are all to be found on the distal parts of the limbs. On the meridians that run through the arms, the points are around and below the elbow, while on those that run through the legs, they are around and below the knee. It is these points that may be used to transfer *qi* to and from the meridian associated with each element. Other points also have specific functions in terms of the transfer of *qi* and particular effects on the meridian in question. These will be mentioned later.

Over the thousands of years that acupuncture has been used in China, two major systems of diagnosis and treatment have developed. One is based entirely on the Law of the Five Elements. The other, while using this law, also diagnoses according to the Eight Principles (sometimes called the Eight Conditions or Eight Syndromes), which I will describe in the next chapter. The fact that there are two systems does not mean that one is wrong and the other right, or even that one is superior to the other. In acupuncture, the diagnosis is more a means to an end than a concrete entity. It is a signpost, indicating to the practitioner which points he should use in order to restore balance to the patient's body energies. Both systems work to restore balance and both are effective in this respect. That they achieve their results by working from different angles is not important.

In this book I am going to concentrate mainly on diagnosis and treatment according to the Eight Principles, since this is the system with which I am more familiar. However, in chapter 7, I quote case histories from both traditions so, before going on to explain the Eight Principles, I shall give a brief outline of the methods of diagnosis used in the Five Elements system.

When a practitioner of the Five Elements system makes a diagnosis, he does so according to the element that is disturbed. A patient is seen as having a susceptibility to injury of a particular element – and this may stem from trauma in childhood or even from when she was still in the womb. Further trauma later in life is therefore likely to affect the meridians related to that element. Once this has occurred, the disturbance may spread to other meridians according to the mother-child and servant-master connections.

The practitioner will treat his patient with the aim of restoring balance among the meridians by removing excess *qi* or stimulating a deficiency of qi. His diagnosis is based on a number of factors such as the patient's colour, his voice, his emotions, and his body odour.

A patient with a disturbance of the Wood element is likely to have a greenish look to her skin, a rancid odour, and a loud aggressive voice. She may be irritable, restless, and unstable, and may be subject to depression.

If the Fire element is affected, the patient will have a red face, a scorched body odour, and a normal or laughing quality of voice. He may have very labile emotions, being up one minute and down the next.

The Earth patient has a yellowish look, a fragrant body odour, and a singing quality to her voice. She may be obsessional, tense and overanxious, and may have a craving for sympathy.

A patient whose Metal meridians are affected will have a white complexion, a rotten smell, and a weeping quality of voice. He is likely to relate his story in grief-laden tones and to regard his problems with a great deal of negativity.

Finally, the Water patient has a bluish look, a putrid smell, and a groaning voice, and she is likely to be timid and fearful.

These, of course, are just the bare bones on which the practitioner bases his diagnosis. In addition, he will also use other methods such as pulse diagnosis (which I shall describe in chapter 5) to confirm which meridians are affected and in which way they are malfunctioning – that is, whether there is an excess or a deficiency. He may then use a variety of points to stimulate or sedate a meridian or to transfer energy from one element to another.

4
CAUSES OF DISEASE

As we have seen, one of the causes of disease, according to traditional Chinese thinking, is invasion by harmful qi. This invasion and its consequent effect on the body has a lot in common with the Western concept of infection and immunity. If the patient's protective *qi* is at a low level, harmful *qi* is able to invade and may overwhelm him because his body is unable to fight back. This is similar to the patient whose immune system is not working at full strength, perhaps because she is taking massive doses of steroids after a transplant operation, or because she has an abnormality of her blood such as leukaemia or, on a less dramatic scale, because she is overtired or has a poor diet. Any of these will lower her resistance to some extent and make her susceptible to infection.

However, in the same way that a particularly virulent infection (such as Covid) can attack healthy people whose immune systems are unimpaired, exceptionally strong harmful *qi* can invade the body even if the protective *qi* is normal. But, in such a case, the protective *qi* will be strong enough to help the body to muster its forces and fight back, enabling the patient to recover. If the protective *qi* is not quite strong enough to fight off the harmful *qi* completely, a balance can develop between the two, resulting in a chronic illness.

But this is not the only way in which illness can arise. It can also be caused from within and, in this case, may be due to emotional upset, inherited factors, or a faulty diet. In the system of acupuncture based on the Eight Principles, there are said to be seventeen major causes of disease – the six eternal factors, the seven emotional factors, and the four miscellaneous factors. In addition to these, disease can be due to trauma, poisoning, or other physical factors.

It is in terms of these causes of disease that the acupuncturist makes his diagnosis. Unlike a Western physician, who will diagnose in terms of which part of the body is diseased and what the abnormality is (for example, inflammation of the appendix, cancer of the lung, cysts in the ovaries and so on), the acupuncturist will make his diagnosis according to what has caused the illness and what effect it has had both on the body's energies and on the function of the *zang-fu* organs. In this chapter we shall look at the effects said to be produced by the seventeen different causative factors.

THE SIX EXTERNAL FACTORS

The six external factors – wind, cold, damp, dryness, heat and summer (or damp) heat – are all forms of harmful qi. Of course, because this form of diagnosis developed in China, these factors originally related to the specific weather conditions prevailing in that part of the world. However, the fact that these were derived in a different climate from our own does not mean that they are invalid in the West, although the frequency of any one type of weather may differ from place to place. Londoners, for example, might be expected to have more illness related to dampness than, say, New Yorkers who, on the other hand, might expect more illness of the summer heat type.

When the Chinese talk about invasion by an external factor, what they mean is an invasion by the essential characteristics of that factor, resulting in a disease that reflects those characteristics. So, you would not expect a patient who has been invaded by cold necessarily to have a lower temperature than normal. Nor does invasion by wind necessarily cause flatulence!

Wind

Wind is said to be prevalent in the spring although, in the West, it is perhaps somewhat more common in the autumn. People are said to be more susceptible to wind diseases if they are exposed to this element when they are hot or have been sweating profusely, or if they have been sleeping in a draught. Wind is predominantly yang, reflecting this in its attributes – it is always moving, insubstantial and agitated, and is often said to attack the upper (yang) part of the body. Wind is thought to enter the body through the pores of the skin, disrupting their functioning so that the patient may sweat excessively. Headache is also a common symptom of diseases caused by wind.

The wind that attacks the patient does not always originate outside the body – it can also develop from within as a result of an excess of *yang* arising in the liver. The symptoms of internally created wind diseases differ somewhat from those produced by external wind. In the former, the complaint might be of ringing in the ears and muscle spasms, together with dizziness and headache. In the latter, the dizziness and headache might be associated with sore throat and a raised temperature.

As already noted, the symptoms of the diseases caused by the external factors usually have the characteristics of those factors. Diseases caused by wind thus tend to have symptoms that, like wind, are constantly changing or moving. A typical case would be a patient with rheumatic fever. Classically, the patient complains of joint pains lasting perhaps no more than a day before they move to another site, and this is combined with fever and sweating. The sweating, as mentioned above, is related to the wind's effect on the pores of the skin, while the fever relates to the *yang* qualities of wind, since *yang* is associated with heat. The patient may also have the headache that is characteristic of wind-induced diseases and – particularly if the disease has been caused by external wind – she may have a dislike of being in a windy place.

Convulsions, spasms and twitches of all types are said to be due to wind, as is facial paralysis which causes a distortion of the features. This latter seems reminiscent of the English folklore cited by mothers who, to stop their children from making faces, tell them, "If the wind changes, you'll get stuck like that".

Cold

The external factor of cold is, of course, prevalent in the winter and is more likely to attack someone if he is not warmly dressed or is exposed to the cold after getting overheated. Cold is a *yin* characteristic so, when it invades, it overwhelms the body's *yang* qi, resulting in an imbalance between *yin* and yang.

The symptoms of disease caused by cold are those you might expect with an excess of *yin* – coldness, slowness, and inhibition of function. The patient may complain of feeling cold and may shiver and look pale. Her feet and hands may be numb or go blue due to poor circulation, and she may have cramps in her muscles. Usually these symptoms are associated with a dislike of the cold.

Invasion of the internal organs by cold, particularly the intestines, may cause diarrhoea and abdominal pain. Cold is also associated with stiffness and stagnation – a sort of 'icing up' of the body. The blood and *qi* are both liable to stagnate in the presence of cold, and the resulting accumulation of either may cause localised pain. So arthritis, in which the patient experiences stiffness and localised areas of pain, may be due to cold. In such cases, the patient may well find that his condition deteriorates during cold weather.

An attack of 'flu in which the patient shivers and complains of aching muscles may also be ascribed to invasion by cold. Fever can occur in cold diseases, but it will not be accompanied by excessive sweating. Frostbite is one condition in which Western medical diagnosis would agree with traditional Chinese medicine that the symptoms – numbness in the feet and hands associated with pallor or blueness – are due to invasion of the body by cold.

Like wind, cold may arise internally. With its *yin* characteristics, it can develop as a result of a weakness in the *yang* of the body, which thus becomes overwhelmed by *yin*. A patient who has a cold disease that has arisen internally is more susceptible to external cold than a healthy person, since she has inadequate *yang* with which to resist it. If she is invaded by external cold, this will exacerbate her condition and may precipitate a crisis.

Damp

Damp in China was said to cause problems mainly in the late summer rainy season. In Japan, as noted in chapter 1, it is a far more frequent cause of illness, occurring all year round. Damp-induced diseases are said to be caused by wearing wet clothes for any length of time or by constantly being in a damp environment.

Damp is described as heavy and stagnant in character, and the diseases that are caused by it have similar characteristics, tending to be long-term problems. The symptoms may include a heavy feeling in the body and the head, and the patient may suffer from dizziness. Swelling of the abdomen or ankles (known, in Western terms, as fluid retention) may occur, and the nose and chest may feel stuffy. Heaviness and chronicity are *yin* characteristics, and therefore damp is predominantly *yin*.

If dampness arises from within, it attacks the *yang* of the spleen and damages it. This can cause chronic digestive problems (since the spleen is considered to be an important digestive organ) and the patient may suffer from recurrent attacks of watery stools or diarrhoea.

Damp causes stagnation and, in the same way that stagnant water is often polluted and smelly, damp is said to cause smelly discharges. Smelly and profuse vaginal discharges, smelly infected urine, and oozing skin conditions are all damp-associated.

When damp attacks the upper part of the body, it produces a heavy feeling in the head, a blocked nose, yellowness of the face, and difficulty in breathing. These symptoms are not unlike those that might appear, according to Western diagnosis, in a patient suffering from Weil's disease which, interestingly enough, is an infection spread by rats living in or near stagnant water, and which is an occupational hazard for sewage workers.

Dryness

In China, diseases caused by dryness are associated with the late autumn – a time that in Europe and the United States is more likely to be associated with damp and wind. Dryness, of course, is said to affect the body's fluids. In Chinese medicine, as in Western, it is recognised as essential that the body fluids be kept in balance. This balance, in Chinese thinking, is intimately associated with the balance of *yin* and yang. Dryness itself is primarily *yang* and therefore can be especially destructive to *yin* fluid, particularly that of the lungs, causing a dry cough associated with a sore throat, and dryness of the mouth and nose.

Dryness may be subdivided into cold dryness and warm dryness. The symptoms of cough and dryness of the throat are common to both, but a patient affected by cold dryness may also have a headache and a dislike of the cold, while a patient whose symptoms are due to warm dryness may be feverish and sweaty.

As you might expect, all dry-skin conditions, such as certain types of dermatitis, are said to be due to dryness. So, too, are wasting diseases in which the patient looks as though he has been literally dried out, like a prune. Tuberculosis, when it affects the lungs, has the characteristics of dryness, being associated with a dry, chesty cough and a general wasting of the body.

Since dryness is *yang* in character, it may develop internally as a result of *yin* deficiency. However, it may also occur if bodily fluids are lost through diarrhoea, vomiting, or excessive sweating, and may thus complicate another disease process.

Heat and summer (or damp) heat

Heat, which is *yang* in character, overwhelms the body's *yin qi* when it invades and upsets the natural balance of *yin* and yang. Summer heat is regarded as being different from heat itself, Chinese summer heat being heavy and damp. Despite the damp element, the *yang* component is strong, and so *yang* symptoms are still produced.

The person who tends to be affected by summer heat is one who remains out in the hot sun for a long time or stays in a room with poor ventilation on a very hot day – the kinds of factors that are known by Western doctors to lead to heatstroke.

Summer heat overwhelms the body's *yin* and injures the body's fluids. It may also affect the mind, causing delirium or coma. Because heat is yang, and because *yang* is associated with acute onsets, the disease may start suddenly. Other symptoms of summer heat include profuse sweating and thirst with fever and restlessness – all *yang* characteristics. Heatstroke, as defined in Western terms, shows all these attributes – thirst, fever and restlessness – and may also affect the patient's level of consciousness.

Although heat itself is yang, a patient may demonstrate *yin* symptoms if he has been drinking large amounts of cold fluids during his exposure to the harmful *qi* of summer heat. In such a case, the symptoms would include a feeling of coldness, headache, abdominal pain and vomiting – the sort of symptoms that, in the West, are usually put down to a summer 'tummy bug'.

Heat itself is usually divided into three degrees of severity – fire (the most severe), heat, and mild heat. Fire can damage the mind, causing loss of consciousness or coma. Heat can combine with some of the other external factors in an invasion of the body, and diseases may be diagnosed as being due to damp heat, dry heat, or heat and wind. In addition, any of the other five external factors may, if very severe, develop into heat and combine heat symptoms with those of their own.

Many diseases that would be diagnosed by Chinese practitioners as due to heat are understood by Western doctors as acute infections, with their common symptoms of fever, thirst, and profuse sweating. Local infections, such as boils or abscesses, are also considered to be heat-induced, since they are red, hot and painful.

When it invades the meridians, heat is said to drive out the blood that circulates there with the *qi* and so may cause haemorrhage. For example, a patient with a severe intestinal infection who was passing bloody stools would be diagnosed as having had her Large Intestine meridian invaded by heat.

Heat can combine with wind to produce severe muscular spasms and convulsions associated with a high fever. If the patient remains untreated, he may finally become delirious and lapse into a coma. Dryness combined with heat will severely affect the lungs and will cause coughing together with spitting of blood. I said earlier that tuberculosis could be ascribed to an invasion by dryness that produces a dry cough and a wasting of the body. At a later stage of the disease, the patient may start to cough up blood. This would be diagnosed as due to heat that developed from the dryness when the latter became increasingly severe. Summer heat may increase in severity and turn into fire, which will exacerbate the symptoms that it has already caused.

THE SEVEN EMOTIONAL FACTORS

Another way in which disease can arise from within is as a result of the seven emotional factors. These can wear away the body's protective qi, leaving the patient defenceless. However, the factors – joy, anger, melancholy, obsessional thinking, grief, fear and fright – have to be very intense or very persistent in order to produce disease. When they are this severe, they often damage the internal organs – anger is said to injure the liver, fright and joy the heart, grief and melancholy the lungs, obsessional thinking the spleen, and fear the kidneys.

In some books, obsessional thinking is referred to as meditation although, of course, obsessional thinking and true meditation are poles apart. It should not be thought that meditation, as practised in many religions, particularly those of Eastern origin, can harm the spleen – or any other organ!

The emotion of anger is predominantly *yang* in character, with *yang* attributes such as suddenness, heat, energy of movement, and the expression of emotions. In addition, its arousal will produce *yang* symptoms similar to those produced by heat.

If the liver – predominantly a *yin* organ – suffers physical damage as a result of an attack by excessive yang, the patient may develop pain and swelling below his ribs on the right side. The liver, in traditional Chinese thought, is responsible for keeping the meridians open and so allowing an unhindered flow of *qi* around the body. It is also thought to be responsible for storing blood. Disruption of its function can thus produce haemorrhage (associated, as we have seen, with heat-induced disease) and menstrual problems. Depression and irritability are also said to result from injury to the liver.

The heart may be damaged by fright – in other words, a sudden, severe shock – or by excessive joy. Either can cause the patient to develop palpitations, anxiety, insomnia and mental disorders, since the heart is the seat of the mind. A Western physician, too, would agree that a sudden shock could cause all these symptoms, although he is unlikely to accept the idea that anxiety, insomnia and mental problems have anything to do with the heart. Still, he would agree that a heart attack could be precipitated in a susceptible person by an extreme shock – or occasionally even by excessive joy and excitement. Patients who have severe angina (intermittent chest pain caused by an inadequate supply of blood to the muscles of the heart) are just as likely to develop pain as a result of watching an exciting football match or meeting up with a long-lost friend as they are from becoming angry or upset.

Fright is a sudden, severe, short-term emotion, while fear is more insidious and long-term and must be persistent in order to produce disease. Fear is said to injure the kidney, which is the seat of willpower. Conversely, if the kidney is deficient in functional *qi* – which is essential for its normal working – the patient is likely to be susceptible to fear.

Injury to the spleen, which is seen as a part of the digestive system, may occur as a result of obsessional thinking or constant worrying. This may cause anorexia (loss of appetite) and a feeling of abdominal distension, especially after meals. Western medicine recognises the mental state of obsessional neurosis in which patients quite commonly number depression and anorexia among their symptoms. Indeed, anorexia nervosa may be thought of as a form of obsession.

Grief and melancholy (the latter including anxiety) are said to affect the lungs and therefore may interfere with breathing. In Western medicine it is known that anxiety may cause hyperventilation or chronic overbreathing, and that patients who suffer from panic attacks can be helped to control them by learning to control their breath.

Anxiety can also be a significant contributory factor to asthmatic attacks in susceptible patients. When hypnotherapy is used to treat asthmatic patients, one of the ways in which it works is to relieve the anxiety that the patient feels at the onset of an attack and so stop the vicious circle in which both anxiety and breathing problems steadily worsen as they feed on each other.

THE FOUR MISCELLANEOUS FACTORS

As well as the external and the emotional factors, disease may be due to four miscellaneous factors. Of these, the first three – irregular eating, excessive stress or lack of physical exercise, and trauma – are also accepted causes of disease in Western medicine, although the symptoms they are said to produce may not be the same. The fourth of the miscellaneous factors is stagnant blood and phlegm.

Irregular eating

'Irregular eating' is a term that includes every form of bad eating habit, such as overeating, undereating, and excessive indulgence in alcohol, fat, or spices. It also includes eating food that is going bad or has been poisoned, and food that has little nutritional value (such as the junk foods so popular in the West).

Overeating is said to interfere with the function of the stomach and the spleen, both of which are intimately concerned in the digestive process. This can cause nausea, vomiting, belching, heartburn, distension, abdominal pain, and diarrhoea. Since food is an important source of qi, undereating can produce a deficiency in the body's qi, causing weakness, dizziness, and emaciation. Unwholesome or poor-quality food will interfere with the function of the stomach and spleen, producing symptoms similar to those caused by overeating. Like Western medicine, Chinese medicine recognises unwholesome food to be a cause of intestinal parasitic diseases. Excessive indulgence in alcohol, fat and spices will stimulate the production of damp heat within the body, which may injure the vital organs. Western doctors would agree that alcohol in excess can damage the liver, while a very fatty diet can damage the heart.

Excessive stress or lack of physical exercise

Long-term stress or overexertion is said to use up the body's protective *qi* and so leave it open to attack by the harmful external factors. It may cause weight loss, exhaustion, dizziness, and palpitations – symptoms also associated with excessive stress in the West. On the other hand, lack of physical exercise can also lower the body's resistance to invasion, since it inhibits the flow of *qi* and blood around the body and can therefore produce symptoms of weakness, exhaustion, shortness of breath and – as recognised in the West – obesity.

Stagnant blood

Stagnant blood is said to have left the blood vessels so it is no longer circulating around the body. Instead, it is retained in the tissues or in body cavities, and it causes symptoms wherever it accumulates. Commonly, it causes pain that may be stabbing or piercing in character, or sometimes colicky (waxing and waning in severity), but the area affected remains constant because the blood, being stagnant, does not move. Haemorrhage (either externally or into the skin) and bruising may also be symptoms of stagnant blood. When haemorrhage occurs, it is usually dark in colour and may contain dark clots, unlike haemorrhage caused by heat, which tends to be a brighter red. Masses, tumours and swelling of the internal organs may also be caused by stagnant blood.

Phlegm

Phlegm – the sticky fluid coughed up from the lungs of people with chest infections – is lumped together with stagnant blood in the list of miscellaneous factors, not because the two conditions necessarily occur together, but because both have stagnant qualities. According to classical Chinese theory, phlegm can affect any part of the body, not just the lungs, and is said to form when the body's use of water is abnormal. Excessive water accumulates within the body and is turned into phlegm, which may invade the organs or the meridians where, because of its stickiness, it may completely block the flow of qi. Such a blockage can be the cause of paralysis coupled with numbness, or with difficulty in speaking and distortion of the face, such as may occur in a patient who has had a stroke. Phlegm may, of course, affect the lungs causing asthma or a severe cough in which the patient brings up large amounts of sputum. It may affect the stomach, producing abdominal distension and allowing fluid to collect in the abdominal cavity. If it attacks the heart – the seat of the mind – its capacity for causing blockages may result in the patient going into a coma. The rattle sometimes heard in the throat of a deeply comatose patient is said to be due to the phlegm lying there. Various soft, movable, superficial lumps – which, in Western medicine, might be diagnosed as cysts or lipomas (fat nodules), for example – are said to be due to accumulations of phlegm under the skin.

THE BASIS OF DIAGNOSIS

A diagnosis in acupuncture must be very exact because the more precise it is, the more likely the treatment is to be successful. Good treatment is based on good diagnosis. A trained acupuncturist will use the four basic techniques put together by Bian Que in the fourth century BCE – observation, listening and smelling, questioning, and pulse diagnosis (the last of these will be covered more fully in the next chapter). Based on this examination, she will be able to decide which causative factor is responsible for the illness and how it has affected the body in terms of the meridians and the organs. On the basis of her findings, she can separate diseases into certain well-defined groups, each associated with one of the Eight Principles. The characteristics associated with individual meridians may indicate which of these is involved in the disease state, and the symptoms may also indicate that certain of the internal, or *zang-fu*, organs have been affected. The way in which the disease has spread through the body from one meridian to another is the province of the Law of the Five Elements, which was covered in the previous chapter.

THE EIGHT PRINCIPLES

The Eight Principles are made up of four pairs of opposites – exterior and interior, cold and hot, *xu* and *shi* (deficiency and excess), and *yin* and yang. The conditions that they cause are sometimes referred to as syndromes (a Western medical term for a collection of symptoms that occur together). The four groups of principles are not mutually exclusive, so it is possible to have, for example, a cold *xu* syndrome or a hot *yang* syndrome.

External and internal refer to the parts of the body that are affected. To a certain extent, they also indicate the severity of the disease, since those that are internal are more serious than those that are external. For example, a skin disease or a mild infection such as a head cold is external, while a disease that attacks the core of the patient's well-being, such as pneumonia, is internal.

Cold and hot refer to the nature of the disease. Cold and hot syndromes exhibit symptoms that are associated with an invasion of the body by cold or by heat.

In a *xu* (deficiency) syndrome, the protective *qi* of the body is deficient and has therefore been powerless to prevent an invasion by harmful qi. In a *shi* (excess) syndrome, however, the protective *qi* is normal but has been overwhelmed by more powerful harmful qi.

External, hot and *shi* syndromes are, by their nature, predominantly *yang* in character, while internal, cold and *xu* syndromes are predominantly yin. However, it is possible to have cold external syndromes, hot internal syndromes, external *xu* syndromes, internal *shi* syndromes, cold *shi* syndromes, and hot *xu* syndromes. Thus, while it is possible to divide all diseases into *yin* types and *yang* types, it is important to remember that *yin* and *yang* are not concrete things but descriptions of the balance between two sides of a whole.

Since external syndromes are predominantly yang, they often develop suddenly and are short lived. Internal syndromes, on the other hand, are more likely to be long term. An external syndrome that is untreated, or against which the body cannot defend itself, may become more severe and move inwards to become an internal syndrome. For example, an elderly or frail person who catches a head cold that then moves into the chest and turns into pneumonia may be seen as suffering from an external syndrome that has become internal. An internal syndrome may also be due to an intrinsic disorder of the internal *zang-fu* organs.

Cold syndromes and hot syndromes, as we have seen, are associated with the sort of symptoms that are caused by invasion by external cold and heat. Cold syndromes, being predominantly yin, are more likely to be long term than hot syndromes, which frequently take the form of acute infections. *Xu* syndromes, too, being 'empty' and therefore yin, are inclined to be long-term compared with the more acute *shi* syndromes.

The concept that an internal syndrome is always more serious than an external one is also found in homoeopathy. Hering's Law of Cure – a homoeopathic creed – states that illness is cured from the top down and from the inside out. So a homoeopath would say that a patient who has eczema and then develops mild asthma is getting worse, even if her eczema has cleared up. However, a patient with asthma who stops having breathing problems is said to be getting better even if he has developed a very severe eczema. The eczema would be seen as an externalisation of his problem, which is an essential step in its cure. Exactly the same is true with acupuncture treatment. A patient who has been suffering from an internal disease may have to trade in her symptoms for those of an external disease before she is finally cured.

In Chinese terms, a common head cold with its symptoms of runny nose, shivering and mild fever could be classified as a cold external syndrome. However, a diagnosis of a cold internal syndrome would be made on a patient who showed signs of coldness, pale skin, diarrhoea, high fever and general prostration – symptoms that, in Western eyes too, would be associated with a far more serious condition, probably produced by a rampant infection.

A hot external syndrome is associated with a slight fever and sweating – the sort of symptoms you might expect to see in a mild case of 'flu. In a hot internal syndrome, however, you would find that the patient has a high fever, severe thirst, restlessness, a flushed face, constipation, and scanty urine. This is the sort of picture you might see in a disease such as scarlet fever, a far more serious condition than 'flu.

Certain types of 'flu that include headache and generalised aching in addition to the mild fever might be diagnosed as external *shi* syndromes. Internal *shi* syndromes, however, present the sort of picture that is associated with a more serious chest infection – congestion in the chest associated with difficulty in breathing, malaise and constipation.

Shi syndromes, with their predominantly *yang* characteristics, are (like external syndromes) usually acute and of sudden onset. They are often associated with fever, flushing of the face, and restlessness. The patient may complain of chest problems, abdominal pain, or difficulty in passing water, all reflecting the excess or 'full' nature of the condition. A kidney infection might be classified as a *shi* syndrome based on symptoms of fever, abdominal pain of sudden onset, and pain on passing water.

Xu syndromes, which are predominantly yin, are inclined to be long standing. They are associated with the sort of symptoms you might expect in a disease where the life force is deficient, such as listlessness, apathy, poor memory, insomnia, shallow breathing and shortness of breath, poor vision, and incontinence. Sadly, these are all symptoms common in elderly, chronically ill patients.

Having ascertained the type of syndrome from which his patient is suffering, the acupuncturist then has to decide which parts of the body are primarily affected. This will be based on his knowledge of the meridians and of the *zang-fu* organs. Symptoms, particularly when localised, may relate to an individual meridian and may be associated with the course of that meridian through the body or with the organ to which it is related. (Symptoms specifically associated with each of the twelve major meridians were mentioned in the previous chapter.)

Certain types of diseases are attributed to disruption, by various factors, of the functioning of the vital organs. It may sound as though this localisation of diagnosis to a meridian or to an organ is akin to the Western practice of diagnosing in terms of a diseased part, but this is not the case. An acupuncture diagnosis does not say that a particular meridian or organ is physically diseased but, rather, that its flow of energy has been disrupted, affecting its function. And the disruption, because it is one of energy, will have an effect not just on the organ or meridian itself but on the whole body.

THE ZANG-FU ORGANS

The functions attributed to the organs by Western medicine, such as the heart's role in the circulation of the blood and the kidney's role in the production of urine, are not the only ones recognised by the Chinese. For them the organs also have other, more subtle, functions in the maintenance of health. The heart, for example, is said to be the seat of the mind or spirit, and disruption of its function will affect the level of consciousness.

Each of the *zang* (solid) organs is linked by one channel to a *fu* (hollow) organ and, by another channel, to a sense organ. Disruption of the *qi* of a *zang* organ can affect the *fu* organ that is related to it. Similarly, the disruption of a *fu* organ's *qi* will have an effect on its associated *zang* organ.

The heart

The heart, which is a *zang* organ, is linked to the small intestine (a *fu* organ) and the tongue (a sense organ). A long illness may affect the heart by causing a general weakness of qi.

If the *qi* of the heart is weak, this will affect the organ's mechanical function, and the heart may develop irregularities in its beat. As a result, the patient may suffer from palpitations and shortness of breath, especially upon exertion – symptoms that the Western physician, too, will associate with heart disease. If the weakness of *qi* is not treated, it may develop into a general deficiency of its active aspect, yang, resulting in yin-associated symptoms such as a lack of energy, coldness, and pallor, together with a susceptibility to other illnesses.

Conversely, a deficiency in the *yin* of the heart may produce symptoms that are due to the relative excess of yang. In this case, the patient may be restless and feverish and have a flushed face. The deficiency of *yin* interferes with the function of the heart and thus of the mind that is housed there. It may cause insomnia, nightmares, poor memory, or other mental symptoms.

A long illness may weaken the heart, in turn interfering with its normal function of pumping blood around the body. A Chinese diagnostician would then say that there was stagnant blood in the heart, which was causing the symptoms and signs demonstrated by the patient – pain in the chest, palpitations, blue lips and blue nails. This corresponds to Western medical thinking to the extent that an orthodox practitioner would recognise these as symptoms of inadequate circulation resulting from poor heart function, although he would not accept the Chinese concept of stagnant blood.

Severe heat, or fire, can also affect the heart. This can arise internally as a result of persistent mental problems that depress the body's *qi* and stimulate the production of fire. The symptoms may include fever (reflecting the causative agent), insomnia (due to the effect on the mind, which is housed in the heart), and problems affecting the tongue, such as ulceration, pain and swelling. The latter are due to fire affecting those parts of the body with which the heart is directly linked.

The liver

The functions of the liver are said to be those of storing blood, maintaining the flow of *qi* around the body, and keeping the tendons in good working order. The *fu* organ to which the liver is linked is the gallbladder (to which it is also linked anatomically). *Qi* runs from the end of the Gall Bladder meridian into the start of the Liver meridian. The sense organ to which the liver is linked is the eye, and it is therefore associated with vision and with the maintenance of normal eyesight.

The functional *qi* of the liver may become depressed, leading to stagnation of *qi* in the Liver meridian. The initial depression of *qi* can arise as a result of mental problems. Stagnant *qi* may go on to produce stagnation of the blood, which may cause menstrual problems.

If the *qi* in the Liver meridian becomes blocked, the patient develops pain below the ribs and in the abdomen, with swelling of the abdomen and sometimes of the breasts. Here again, there is a link with Western medical diagnosis, since patients who are diagnosed with cirrhosis of the liver not uncommonly have ascites (swelling of the abdomen due to an accumulation of fluid) together with gynaecomastia (swelling of the breasts).

Severe heat, or fire, affecting the liver can be due to an overindulgence in alcohol or to excessive smoking. It may also be secondary to depression of the liver's qi. The fire prevents *qi* from flowing normally and, as a result, the patient may suffer from dizziness, headache and irritability, and may develop an inflammation of the eyes. If the blood stored by the liver becomes affected by fire, haemorrhage may result, manifesting as nosebleeds or as vomiting of blood.

Heat can be associated with wind in an attack on the liver. In this case, the symptoms produced are attributable to both these external factors. The patient develops a high fever and may have convulsions, possibly associated with neck rigidity and, later, coma. These are symptoms recognised in Western medicine as being due to an infection affecting the central nervous system – meningitis or encephalitis.

Cold may affect the liver and cause stagnation of qi, particularly in the Liver meridian itself. This causes abdominal pain and, if the patient is male, can produce swelling and pain in the testicles, since the meridian runs through this area.

The liver is seen as a storehouse for blood, so chronic disease or haemorrhage, which are said to use up those stores, will produce a deficiency. As a result, the body is no longer adequately nourished. Other functions of the liver will also be affected. There may be spasms in the tendons and muscles, which depend on the liver for their normal function, and the patient may have disturbances of vision, such as blurring and dizziness, and her eyes may feel dry and gritty. If the patient is female, her menstrual cycle can be affected, with her periods becoming scanty and irregular.

The spleen

The spleen is credited by the Chinese with control of digestion. It is said to be responsible for the proper absorption of nutrients from the ingested food and for their distribution around the body, so it is intimately linked with the stomach and its functions.

As we saw in chapter 2, the beginning of the Spleen meridian follows on from the end of the Stomach meridian and receives *qi* directly from it. The sense organ to which the spleen is linked is the mouth (although, as already mentioned, the tongue is associated with the heart). The spleen is also said to control the blood, ensuring that it remains within the blood vessels, and to be responsible for the maintenance of healthy muscles.

Because the spleen is involved in the extraction of *qi* from food, it will naturally be affected by our eating habits. Irregular eating will cause the spleen's functional *qi* to be weakened. Such a weakness may also be due to chronic stress or to long-term illness which has given rise to a poor appetite and consequent inadequate food intake.

If its own functional *qi* is weak, the spleen will be unable to extract *qi* adequately from what little food is being eaten, so that a vicious circle is set up. The patient develops lassitude, a sallow complexion, and diarrhoea due to the overall deficiency of body nutrition. The muscles are no longer maintained in good condition, so the body loses its firmness. As a result, prolapse of the uterus or rectum (back passage) may occur. Blood is not properly contained within the blood vessels, which may result in spontaneous bruising or haemorrhage.

Because of its intimate association with the stomach and digestion, the spleen is susceptible to injury from any form of unbalanced diet. If excessive amounts of raw or cold food are eaten, this may open the spleen to attack from cold and damp. Again, this will be associated with poor appetite, and the patient may develop abdominal pain and diarrhoea. Because cold is inclined to cause stagnation, the flow of *qi* may become blocked and cause swelling in the upper abdomen, associated with lassitude and a heavy feeling in the head.

The lungs

The lungs are, naturally, in charge of respiration. In addition to bringing oxygen into the body and expelling carbon dioxide, respiration takes in clean *qi* and gets rid of waste qi. The lungs are also said to control the use of water in the body and to maintain the health of the skin and the hair.

The Lung meridian is coupled in the 24 hour cycle with one of the other water-controlling meridians, the Urinary Bladder, so that when one is at its highest point in terms of the flow of qi, the other is at its lowest. The lungs also link with the large intestine (since *qi* flows from the Lung meridian into the Large Intestine meridian). The sense organ with which it is connected is, of course, the nose.

Chronic lung disease from whatever cause may result in a deficiency of the lung's yin. This affects the lung's control of the body's water and results in a dry mouth, fever, night sweats, and a dry cough, sometimes with some blood being coughed up. In Western terms, these are all symptoms that may be associated with a diagnosis of tuberculosis. I mentioned earlier that the symptoms of tuberculosis could be produced by an invasion of the lungs by heat and dryness – both predominantly *yang* factors whose long-term presence can result in a chronic deficiency of yin.

The lungs can also be affected by wind, which may be accompanied by cold. The wind produces a cough and a blocked nose, while the additional cold may aggravate the condition, causing a sensation of coldness, a nasal discharge, and the coughing up of sputum. These are symptoms that are often associated with the common cold. If the invading wind is accompanied by heat, the symptoms are those of a rather more severe form of the infection, with fever, sore throat, and purulent nasal discharge and sputum.

If the body's use of water – controlled by the lungs – becomes disrupted, fluid can accumulate within the lungs as damp or phlegm. This, in turn blocks the flow of qi, and the patient becomes short of breath and brings up a lot of white sputum. Phlegm may also develop as a result of the invasion of the lungs by wind and heat. This, too, will block the flow of *qi* so that the patient develops a cough with shortness of breath. In this case, because the phlegm is hot, blood stagnates; as a result, the sputum that is brought up is not only copious but also purulent.

The kidneys

As well as having a role in maintaining the body's water balance, the kidneys are said to be in charge of reproduction, growth, and development. Although these last three are not functions associated with the kidneys in Western medicine, it is interesting to note that they may be associated with the adrenal glands which are situated immediately above the kidneys on the back wall of the abdominal cavity. The adrenals produce steroid hormones, and disruption of their function may produce abnormalities of growth and development, as well as interfering with normal reproduction. The adrenals also secrete the hormones that regulate the kidneys' function of excreting water.

In Chinese medicine, the kidneys work together with the lungs in their capacity of controlling the body's use of water. The kidneys are also said to regulate the distribution around the body of clean qi, extracted from the inhaled air by the lungs. They are responsible for the formation of the bone marrow, the blood, and the brain, which is considered a specialised form of marrow. They are linked to the bladder (as they are anatomically) since the end of the Urinary Bladder meridian opens into the start of the Kidney meridian. The sense organ with which they are associated is the ear, and deafness in the elderly is said to be due to a deficiency of functional *qi* in the kidneys.

Long-term illness can weaken the kidneys' qi. Such weakness may also occur congenitally, or it may be due to senility. Whatever the cause, symptoms associated with urination are likely to occur, including an increase in frequency, dribbling or incontinence. The reproductive system may be affected, resulting in infertility. Because the kidneys are associated with and work together with the lungs, weakness of their functional *qi* may also cause shortness of breath or asthma.

A deficiency of *yin* or yang, either of which may occur as the result of a long illness, may have an effect on the kidneys. It is said that such a deficiency can also be due to an overindulgence in sexual activity. If *yin* is deficient, the patient may experience dizziness, blurring of vision, poor memory, and tinnitus (ringing in the ears) due to the kidneys' inability to maintain the normal functions of the brain and of the ears. Since a deficiency of *yin* necessarily results in a relative excess of yang, yang-type symptoms such as feverishness and night sweats will occur.

The association of *yang* with activity means that a deficiency of *yang* in the kidneys will lead to a reduction in the activity of the kidneys. This can cause fluid retention and reduced production of urine. The reduction in activity may also affect bladder function, resulting in problems such as dribbling and retention of urine. In addition, the relative excess of *yin* will cause pallor and symptoms of coldness and male patients may become impotent.

The pericardium

The pericardium may be invaded by heat. This will produce symptoms of high fever, delirium, and coma as a result of the effect on the mind, which is housed in the heart.

The gallbladder

Jaundice is said to be caused by an invasion of the gallbladder by damp heat. This may be due to a primary malfunction in the liver or to long-term overindulgence in alcohol or rich food. Because damp causes stagnation, the flow of qi is impaired. The resulting blockage prevents bile from being excreted freely. Thus the patient develops jaundice and may vomit bile. It is the blockage of *qi* in the gallbladder and the liver that produces the pain many jaundiced patients experience in the upper right part of their abdomens.

The stomach

Overeating may disrupt the functional *qi* of the stomach, causing food to be retained within it. This will result in distension and pain in the upper abdomen, together with belching, nausea and vomiting.

Ingesting large amounts of raw or cold food may cause the stomach to be attacked by cold. This can also occur if the patient gets soaked by cold rain. The invading cold causes stagnation of the functional *qi* of the stomach, resulting in the retention of fluid and causing pain and swelling in the upper abdomen and, sometimes, vomiting. Similar symptoms may also be due to depression of the stomach's yang, which may occur after a long illness. The deficiency of active yang, together with a relative excess of yin, are the factors that cause the stagnation in this case. Eating large quantities of rich food can cause heat to accumulate in the stomach, resulting in a burning pain in the upper abdomen, thirst, vomiting, and bad breath.

The large intestine

Although it lies further along the digestive tract than the stomach, the large intestine may also have its function disrupted by dietary abnormalities. Eating excessive amounts of raw, cold or unwholesome food may cause the large intestine to be affected by damp heat. The damp causes stagnation and thus hinders the normal flow of qi. As a result, the patient develops diarrhoea and abdominal pain. The heat may cause haemorrhage, which shows itself as blood in the stools. These are symptoms that Western doctors, too, would associate with food poisoning.

Disruption of the flow of *qi* in the large intestine may also be due to stagnation of the blood flow, causing constipation, abdominal pain, and distension. A more serious version of this may be caused by an invasion of the large intestine by heat due to overeating or to a particular susceptibility of the patient to weather changes. This can cause inflammation of the intestine and the formation of abscesses in addition to the symptoms already mentioned.

The bladder

Damp heat may invade the bladder and cause the sort of symptoms that are associated in Western medicine with infections of the urinary tract, including frequent passing of water with associated burning and pain. The heat can also cause haemorrhage and consequent passage of blood in the urine. If the condition is not treated, the damp may give rise to stagnation which, in turn, may result in the formation of stones.

5

METHODS OF DIAGNOSIS

The experienced acupuncturist's familiarity with the functions of the meridians and of the *zang-fu* organs will enable him to assess which of these has had its flow of *qi* disrupted and in what manner. However, he will also use pulse and tongue diagnosis to decide how this disruption has been brought about and, in addition, may look at the patient's face, skin and general appearance and ask her about her eating and sleeping habits, urine and bowels. From all of this, the acupuncturist will be able to determine whether the patient is suffering from a *xu* (deficiency) syndrome or a *shi* (excess) syndrome, whether *yin* or *yang* is predominant, and which of the external, emotional or miscellaneous factors may be responsible for the illness.

THE PULSE

The radial artery, which runs across the wrist, is used by both Chinese and Western physicians when they take a pulse, but their methods are quite different. Chinese pulse diagnosis is a very exact science, far removed from the simple counting of beats and assessment of rhythm practised in the West, and it may take a student many years of practice before he is proficient at it. This is why students who have only attended short courses in acupuncture will usually rely mainly on the condition of the tongue to back up their diagnosis.

Tongue diagnosis will give the same indications as pulse diagnosis, and has the advantage that it is much easier to learn. However, it is not nearly as accurate. The difference between a practitioner using only tongue diagnosis and one who combines this with pulse diagnosis may be compared to the difference between two Western doctors, one armed with a stethoscope and blood pressure measuring equipment and the other with an electrocardiogram (ECG) machine as well. The first doctor can quite easily diagnose a patient who has had a heart attack from the symptoms that are presented and from the signs that he can observe using his equipment. However, the doctor with the ECG machine will be able to tell which part of the heart has been affected and how severe the heart attack has been. He will also be able to monitor, on an hour-to-hour basis, any improvement or deterioration in his patient's condition

When a Western physician takes a pulse, she puts her fingers lightly on one of the patient's wrists and feels the radial artery somewhere along the stretch where it runs just under the skin. A Chinese physician, while using the same stretch of the same artery, will feel it at six well-defined places on each wrist, three superficial and three deep. Each of these pulses reflects the condition of one of the twelve major meridians and their associated organs, allowing their balance to be assessed, while the character of the pulse as a whole indicates the type of syndrome affecting the patient. Comparing each pulse against the others allows any sign of excess or deficiency in a particular meridian to be detected.

All the superficial pulses are associated with the *fu* (hollow) organs and their meridians, which are predominantly yang. On the right wrist are the pulses that are linked to the large intestine, stomach, and *sanjiao*, while on the left are those linked to the small intestine, gallbladder and urinary bladder.

The deep pulses are associated with the *zang* (solid) organs which are predominantly *yin* – the lung, spleen and pericardium on the right, and the heart, liver and kidney on the left.

However, this is not the end of the story where *yin* and *yang* are concerned. Left-sidedness is associated with *yin* and right-sidedness with yang, so all the pulses on the left wrist reflect the total *yin* of the body and all those on the right wrist the total yang. If all the pulses on the right are normal but those on the left are stronger, this indicates an excess of yin, while the reverse indicates an excess of yang. Similarly, normal pulses on the right combined with weak pulses on the left suggest a deficiency of yin, while a deficiency of *yang* would present as normal pulses on the left and weak pulses on the right.

We have already seen that the aspects of *yin* and *yang* are not concrete but fluctuate according to how you look at them. This applies just as much to pulse diagnosis as to anything else. An outer or exterior position is always predominantly *yang* compared to an inner position, which is predominantly yin. The outer pulses are those that are closest to the wrist (and therefore furthest from the heart), while the inner pulses are those slightly higher up the arm.

If the outer pulses (relating to the large intestine and lung on the right, the small intestine and heart on the left) are stronger than the inner pulses (*sanjiao* and pericardium on the right, urinary bladder and kidney on the left), this indicates a relative excess of *yang* in the body. If, however, the inner pulses are stronger, a relative excess of *yin* is indicated. The balance of *yin* and *yang* can also be determined by comparing the superficial and the deep pulses, since deepness is *yin* while superficiality is yang.

Having determined the balance of *yin* and *yang* and the balance of *qi* in the organs and meridians, the acupuncturist will then assess the quality of the pulse in order to elicit further information as to the type of syndrome affecting the patient. Numerous qualities of pulse have been described, although many of these categories appear to run into each other and their fine distinctions are perceived only by the expert. However, for our purposes, they may be divided into a few broadly based groups.

The first of these is the rapid pulse, which is defined as having more than five beats to a breath (note that, in Chinese medicine, the pulse is timed by the patient's breathing and not by the doctor's watch). A rapid pulse often occurs when there is an excess of *yang* and therefore increased activity in the body, or when the patient is suffering from a hot syndrome. This tallies with Western diagnosis, in which a rapid pulse (albeit timed by the clock) may be associated with a fever.

The rapid pulse may be either forceful or weak, a forceful quality indicating an excess of *qi* or a *shi* syndrome, whereas a weak pulse would be indicative of a *xu* (deficiency) syndrome.

There is, as you would expect, a strong correlation between the Chinese concept of a normal pulse rate – between four and five beats to the breath – and that held by physicians in the West. In the West, where the pulse is measured as number of beats per minute, the norm is around seventy two, while the normal number of breaths per minute is around sixteen. Divide the normal pulse rate by the normal breath rate and you come up with four and a half, the midway point of the Chinese normal range.

If an excess or deficiency of *qi* occurs without the involvement of cold or heat, as in a *shi* or *xu* syndrome, this can also be diagnosed from the pulse. A *xu* pulse feels weak when pressed lightly and disappears completely on heavy pressure, whereas a *shi* pulse feels forceful no matter whether you press lightly or firmly. A thready pulse may also indicate a *xu* syndrome, while a large bounding pulse may occur in a *shi* syndrome.

External and internal syndromes also have their own diagnostic types of pulse. External syndromes may be indicated, in the early stages, by a superficial or floating pulse. This is a pulse that is readily felt when the pressure exerted is light but it becomes weak if pressed hard. It gives a sensation of floating on the surface of the skin. A fine distinction of this type of pulse is one that conveys the floating feeling and yet is either weak or forceful. If it is weak, it suggests that the patient is suffering from a long-term illness and a deficiency of yang. A forceful floating pulse, however, would be associated with an external syndrome in which there was an excess of yang.

A deep pulse is the diagnostic opposite of a floating pulse. It is necessary to exert increased pressure in order to feel this pulse, which is associated with internal syndromes. Again, it may be forceful or weak, force being associated with an excess and weakness with a deficiency.

Sometimes a pulse is described as being slippery or gliding, feeling almost as though it is wriggling under the fingers and often compared to ball bearings rolling on a plate. This type of pulse is an indication that phlegm is causing problems. When the pulse is forceful, it suggests that the seat of the patient's problem is in the digestive tract. When it is weak, it indicates that phlegm has accumulated due to a general weakness of the body. A full, gliding pulse may also occur in healthy people, however, particularly in women during pregnancy.

A completely different quality of pulse, with none of the easy movement of the slippery pulse, is known as a rough pulse. It may occur in conditions of deficiency of *qi* or of blood, particularly if the kidney is affected, in which case it will be weak. Or it may also indicate stagnation due to an invasion by cold damp, in which case it will be forceful.

An irregular pulse in Western medicine indicates an irregular heartbeat due to an electrical misfiring in the mechanism that regulates the contraction of the heart muscle. To a Chinese physician, it is an indication of stagnation of blood with interference to the flow of *qi* and a deficiency of yang.

The bowstring or wiry pulse is hard and forceful, giving the impression of a tightly pulled string. While it may be found in a healthy person, it can also occur in a patient who is in pain or in one who has a deficiency of *yin* with a relative excess of *yang* in the liver.

Within these definitions, there are further divisions. For example, as well as the slow and rapid categories, varieties of rate and rhythm may be described as knotted, intermittent, scattered, moving, hasty, slowing or fast.

THE TONGUE

Although tongue diagnosis has fewer nuances than pulse diagnosis and takes less time to learn, it is still of great value to the experienced practitioner of Chinese medicine. In Western medicine a healthy tongue is said to be pink and moist with little or no coating. This is also accepted as normal in Chinese medicine, but assessment of the tongue goes much further than this. As with the pulse, the findings are expressed in terms of the cause of the patient's disease and the energy imbalances that have resulted.

A normal tongue is pink. Anything else is said to be abnormal. Abnormal colours are classified as pale, red, purplish-red, or purple. A pale tongue, as you might guess, is indicative of a deficiency syndrome (particularly a deficiency of yang) or of a disease caused by cold. A deficiency of blood will also cause a pale tongue, which tallies with the Western acceptance of a pale tongue as one of the signs of anaemia. If the tongue appears glossy and pale, it suggests that the problem is a long-standing one.

If the patient has a wet pale tongue, this indicates that the *yang* of the spleen is deficient. According to the Law of the Five Elements, the spleen is the master of the kidney. If the spleen is deficient (the paleness indicating deficiency), then it will be unable to control the kidney. This will affect the body's fluids, causing the tongue to become abnormally wet.

A red tongue is suggestive of a disease caused by heat or of a deficiency of yin, causing a relative excess of yang. A purplish-red tongue occurs in acute diseases caused by heat, such as acute fevers. In such cases the tongue may also be dry, indicating that the body's fluids have been affected by the heat. A purplish-red tongue can also occur in patients who, due to a prolonged and severe illness, are deficient in yin. In such a case it is likely to have a glossy appearance, signifying that there has been damage to both the *yin* and the body's fluids.

A purple tongue is recognised by Western doctors as being associated with heart disease, and particularly with heart failure and inadequate pumping of the blood around the body. In Chinese medicine it may indicate stagnation of *qi* and of blood. It may also occur if there is an excess of internal cold due to a deficiency of yang.

The coating of the tongue is said to be formed from food residues together with *yang qi* derived from the spleen, and so it will reflect any abnormalities of the digestive system. Its colour and condition are also indicative of various states occurring within the body. The coating may be described as white, yellow, greyish-black, or peeled. In addition, it may be thin, thick, sticky, moist or dry. A thick coating usually indicates a more serious problem than a thin coating of the same colour. Patchy coating occurs when the spleen and stomach are not working together properly in the production of qi. Moistness is suggestive of an invasion by damp, or of an imbalance in the body's fluids due to a deficiency in the *yang* of the kidney or spleen (its master according to the Law of the Five Elements). A dry coating is usually due to a deficiency of bodily fluids following an invasion by heat, and a sticky coating suggests that phlegm is the cause of the patient's condition.

A thin white coating may occur in a healthy person but, when seen in a patient suffering from a disease, it indicates an invasion of the lungs by wind and cold. A thin yellow coating, on the other hand, is never normal and may mean that the lungs have been invaded by wind and heat.

If the coating of the tongue is white and thick, it suggests that food is being retained. A more serious and long-term form of this is suggested by a thick yellow coating.

A sticky white coating indicates invasion by cold and damp or the retention within the body of phlegm and damp. It might be seen, for example, in a patient with bronchitis. A sticky yellow coating indicates retention of damp heat or a blockage in the lungs caused by phlegm and heat, and might be seen in a patient suffering from a lung abscess.

A dry white coating to the tongue indicates invasion by a pestilential factor – a term used to include all forms of epidemic contagious diseases. A dry yellow coating reflects both heat and an imbalance of bodily fluids, suggesting an accumulation of heat in the stomach and intestines that has damaged *yin* and fluids.

A yellow coating may, of course, also be seen on the tongues of smokers, so an acupuncturist will always want to know whether or not the patient smokes. His pleasure on hearing that a patient is a non-smoker will be twofold. Firstly, it will make his diagnosis easier, because the colour of the tongue and its coating will not be masked. And, secondly, his treatment will not be counteracted by the patient continuing to assault his body with toxins!

The tongue may sometimes have a bald or peeled appearance. This is often associated, in Western terms, with a severe vitamin deficiency. To the Chinese physician, it may indicate a prolonged and severe illness in which the patient's protective *qi* has been severely damaged and a considerable deficiency of *yin* has occurred – events that might be associated with malnutrition.

A moist, greyish-black coating on the tongue usually suggests that cold and damp have been retained within the body or that inner cold has welled up due to a deficiency of *yang* and a relative excess of yin. A greyish-black coating that is dry and seen on a red tongue indicates a drying out of bodily fluids by excessive heat which, in turn, may be due to a deficiency of *yin* with a relative excess of yang. This sort of tongue may occur in patients who, in Western terms, are dehydrated.

The tongue can, of course, be coloured by things other than disease and smoking. Sweets, soft drinks, red wine, and some fruits and vegetables can all stain the tongue, so it is important to ensure that you haven't dyed your tongue a new shade when you go to see your acupuncturist!

In addition to its colour, the condition of the tongue can reveal important things to the practitioner about her patient's condition. A patient with a large and flabby tongue that is pale, and perhaps shows indentations from his teeth around the edge, is likely to be suffering from a general deficiency of *qi* and *yang* and to have an accumulation within his body of phlegm and damp. If the tongue is flabby and red, this suggests an excess of heat that is affecting the stomach or the heart. A flabby purplish-red tongue occurs when there is stagnation of blood. A tongue that is a normal shade of pink may also be flabby – in this case, it would suggest an accumulation of damp heat in the spleen or stomach, or a deficiency of yang.

A tongue that has fissures in it and looks cracked may be normal in some people so, if your tongue looks like this, you may be asked whether it has always looked so. If, however, the cracks have only appeared with the onset of the illness, they may indicate a drying up of the body's fluids due to excessive heat, and a deficiency of *yin* in the kidney, with a relative excess of yang.

The tongue may display little bumps on its surface. These are usually red and suggest excessive heat with a drying up of bodily fluids, and may also indicate stagnation of blood. This appearance is described as a thorny tongue and it may be seen in a patient who has recently suffered from an infectious illness. White bumps on the tongue or flat purple blotches may occur in severe cases of invasion by heat, and the latter may also indicate stagnation of blood and qi.

A stiff and tremulous tongue is usually associated in Western medicine with some form of neurological disorder. In Chinese medicine it is an indication of a disturbance of the mind caused by phlegm and heat. The tongue is, of course, the sense organ that is linked to the heart, which is the seat of the mind. A stiff, tremulous tongue may also be seen in a patient suffering from a *yin* deficiency in the liver due to invasion by heat, or it may be associated with an obstruction of the collateral channels by wind and phlegm. When it is seen during a prolonged illness, it suggests an overall deficiency of *qi* and of *yin*. A tongue that is deviated to one side of the mouth, such as may occur after a stroke, is also said to indicate obstruction of the collateral channels by wind and phlegm. Wind is often said to be the causative factor of a stroke.

Wind can cause blockages that interfere with both movement and sensation, so if a patient complains that his tongue feels numb, it may indicate that wind is a causative factor in his illness. This may have arisen either from a *yin* deficiency or, if the tongue is red, from an excess of *qi* affecting the liver.

A thin tongue is said to indicate a deficiency syndrome. If the tongue is pale this suggests that the deficiency is one of *qi* and of blood whereas, if it is red, the deficiency is likely to be of yin, producing a relative excess of yang.

If while examining the patient's tongue, the acupuncturist becomes aware of bad breath, this is an indication that heat is affecting the stomach.

Tongue diagnosis and pulse diagnosis are the two most valuable diagnostic tools available to the acupuncturist, which is why I have gone into the details of both techniques before mentioning any others. When you visit an acupuncturist, however, it is likely that your general appearance will be observed and that you'll be asked questions about yourself before any reference is made to your pulse or tongue.

HABITS AND OTHER SYMPTOMS AND SIGNS

In both Western and Chinese medicine, the patient's habits may provide clues as to the problem affecting her and its cause. But the interpretation that an acupuncturist puts on the information that the patient provides will be quite different from that made by a Western physician. For example, a patient who has to stand a great deal in the course of her work may develop problems affecting the kidney and its meridian, while a patient who sits all day may have problems affecting the spleen. The spleen may also be affected by excessive concentration (a lesser degree of the obsessional thinking mentioned earlier), as may the stomach, with which it works in the digestion of food and extraction of qi. You may see this sort of effect in someone who is a workaholic who spends long hours at his desk, striving for perfection in his work, and ends up developing a peptic ulcer.

Eating habits

The patient's eating habits are important, too, as are her reactions to food. As we have seen, overeating or the consumption of junk foods may contribute to the development of disease, as may an excessive intake of spices, fat or alcohol.

If a patient feels better after she has eaten, this suggests that she is deficient in *qi* – it is the *qi* derived from the food she has just eaten that is giving her this temporary relief. Conversely, a patient whose symptoms increase in severity after he has eaten is likely to have an excess of qi, with the *qi* in the food making matters worse. If he feels bloated after eating, this suggests that the *qi* he has extracted from the food is being prevented from circulating correctly and that there is stagnation. Constant thirst indicates a hot syndrome, while an absence of thirst suggests an invasion by cold or damp.

Tastes

Certain tastes are associated with certain elements. So, when they appear abnormally, they may indicate problems relating to the organs or meridians linked to those elements.

A sour taste is associated with Wood, a bitter taste with Fire, sweetness with Earth, a spicy taste with Metal, and saltiness with Water. So a salty taste in the mouth may be a symptom of disturbance of the kidney (one of the Water organs) by heat. Since the spleen is associated with Earth, damp heat affecting the spleen may produce a sweet taste in the mouth. Heat affecting the Fire-related heart is likely to result in a bitter taste. A patient who has lost his sense of taste altogether is likely to have a deficiency of his spleen's functional qi.

Sleeping patterns

A patient's illness may also be reflected in his sleeping patterns. Excessive sleepiness may be due to a deficiency of *yang* with a corresponding excess of the inactive principle, yin. Insomnia, on the other hand, may indicate a deficiency of *yin* in the liver and kidney or an overall deficiency of qi. Early morning waking suggests a deficiency of qi, particularly in the Gall Bladder meridian, or it may be due to an excess of heat in the heart. The heart and gallbladder are also implicated if the patient is a very light sleeper, when a disturbance of the *qi* of either may be involved.

Urine and bowels

Like a Western physician, an acupuncturist may ask about the patient's urine and bowels. Here again, though, the conclusions drawn from the answers will be different from the Western ones.

If the patient passes a lot of urine or has to get up at night to pass water, he is likely to have a deficiency in the kidney's yang. A total deficiency of *qi* in the kidney and bladder, however, may reduce the amount of urine produced to below normal. Incontinence may also be caused by a deficiency of the kidney's functional qi.

Blood in the urine may be an indication of damp heat in the bladder, heat being a common cause of haemorrhage. If the urine is a particularly dark yellow in colour, this also suggests an invasion by heat, whereas pale urine indicates an invasion by cold or a deficiency of the kidney's yang, with a relative excess of yin.

The type of stools that the patient passes may indicate the state of her intestines. Since damp is associated with stagnation and smelly discharges, the passage of watery, smelly stools is a good indication that the intestines have been invaded by damp heat.

Eyes

Red and painful eyes may indicate that the patient is suffering from an excess of *yang* and heat. If they itch, an invasion by wind and heat may have occurred. The organ with which the eyes are linked is the liver. If the kidney's *yin* is deficient and, as a result, it fails to nourish the liver (its child according to the Law of the Five Elements), the *yin* of the latter may also become deficient. This may be suspected if a patient complains that light hurts his eyes. A deficiency of *qi* in the kidney, resulting in a deficiency in the liver, may produce double vision. Blurred vision, however, can be a result of an abnormality of the blood or of yin.

Observations

While the acupuncturist is interviewing the patient he will, like any Western physician, be observing him. If the patient appears apprehensive – or, at least, more apprehensive than might be considered normal for a patient on his first visit to an acupuncturist – this may suggest a problem with the kidney or urinary bladder or their meridians. The kidney and urinary bladder may also be involved if the patient is overweight or has abnormally cold hands.

If the patient is tense, the liver and gallbladder may be implicated, while a patient whose attention wanders may have problems with the spleen or stomach.

A great deal can be discovered by observing the patient's face. As with the tongue, the colour can be very informative. A red face, of course, is suggestive of an invasion by heat. A sallow complexion indicates a deficiency, usually affecting the spleen (which is responsible for the extraction and circulation of qi) and also suggests an invasion by damp. Damp heat in the spleen may produce a dark, orange-coloured jaundice, while a lighter yellow jaundice may be due to damp cold.

A very pale complexion, too, may be associated with a total body deficiency of *qi* or of *yang* (such as might occur after a haemorrhage), or with a deficiency of *qi* together with cold in the lungs. If the patient's face is pale but her cheeks and lips are red, a deficiency of *yin* may have resulted in the production of heat through the relative excess of yang.

Pale lips, like a pale complexion, signify a deficiency, particularly in the lungs. Bright red lips, on the other hand, are indicative of heat, especially affecting the heart. Dry lips suggest that heat is affecting the spleen or that there is an imbalance of the body's fluids. The condition of the spleen is also implicated if the lips are swollen.

There are differing views as to the diagnostic value of lines and blemishes in various positions on the face. Some practitioners believe that the entire body is reflected in the face. Others, however, dispute the reliability of this type of diagnosis.

The condition of the skin and nails is more widely accepted as useful in diagnosis. Dry, flaky skin suggests that the circulation of *qi* and blood is sluggish, leaving the skin inadequately nourished. If the skin becomes puffy, this may be due to a blockage in the flow of qi, while a deficiency of *qi* will result in the skin becoming thin and wrinkled.

Nails that break easily or seem soft also suggest a deficiency of *qi* or blood, particularly one affecting the liver (upon whose normal function the health of the nails depends).

Although the techniques of acupuncture and the ways in which diagnoses are made are so different from those used in Western medicine, a patient who visits an acupuncturist for the first time may well feel that his initial consultation was rather similar to one he might have had with his own family doctor. Many of the questions asked will be the same, and examinations of tongue, pulse, skin and nails will have a familiar ring. And, although Chinese and Western doctors will interpret the symptoms and signs presented to them very differently, in both cases it is on this interpretation and diagnosis that treatment will be based.

6

METHODS OF TREATMENT

In Western medicine, both diagnosis and treatment are usually based upon a part of the body. For example, a diagnosis of a broken bone will be followed by treatment of that bone by putting it in a splint, and a diagnosis of an irregular heartbeat will be followed by treatment of the heart with drugs to regulate its rhythm. A patient diagnosed with gallstones is likely to have her gallbladder removed and, with it, the stones. However, removing a patient's gallstones does not treat their initial cause. While the stones do not re-form, since the gallbladder is no longer there, the imbalance that originally created them has not been cured by the operation.

In Chinese medicine, the aim of treatment is not just to alleviate the illness itself but to do so by removing its cause. A patient whose illness is diagnosed as being due to invasion by heat, no matter what his symptoms may be, will be given treatment aimed as dispelling heat from his body. Similarly, if a patient is diagnosed with excessive *yin*, the treatment will be focused on sedating *yin* and stimulating *yang*. It is, of course, sometimes possible to treat specific symptoms with acupuncture, since some acupuncture points have specific effects – to lower blood pressure, for example, or to stop vomiting. However, these points are not usually used as a complete treatment in themselves.

Acupuncture, like many other complementary therapies, is a way of restoring the body's energy flow to a normal state so that the body can get on with the work of healing itself. When there is a deficiency of *qi*, *yin*, or *yang*, the system must be stimulated. When there is an excess, it must be reduced. Heat, cold, wind, damp, dryness, or phlegm must be eliminated from the body, and stagnant blood must be set flowing again. Imbalances among the meridians must be remedied by sending *qi* into a deficient meridian from one that has excess. A mother meridian must be encouraged to nourish its child, and a master meridian must be adjusted so that it has appropriate control over its servant. If there is a blockage of *qi* flowing along the course of a single meridian, this must be unblocked.

Each meridian's points have specific functions relating to the transfer of energy. The element points have already been mentioned in chapter 3. In addition, each meridian has a source point by which it is linked to its organ. Thus, the source point on the Lung meridian can be used to treat the lung itself, while that on the Kidney meridian can be used to treat the kidney, and so on. Some points are specific for dispelling the various external factors – heat, wind, cold, damp, dryness and summer heat. Others have particular effects on *yin* or *yang*, either stimulating or sedating. On each of the major meridians – except that of the heart – there are one or more intersection or meridian connection points by which that meridian is linked to others. These points are useful for the treatment of conditions in which several meridians are affected.

Along the Urinary Bladder meridian, as it runs down the back, there is a series of points that have an effect on the other major meridians. These are known as the associated or shu points. Each meridian is related to one shu point lying between UB 13 and UB 28, parallel to the spine. On the front of the trunk are twelve similar alarm or mu points, each of which is also connected to one of the major meridians. However, the mu points don't lie on a single meridian. Six of them (those relating to the Pericardium, Heart, Stomach, Sanjiao, Small Intestine, and Urinary Bladder meridians) are midline and are points on the Ren meridian (or Vessel of Conception). The others are bilateral. The Lung mu point, the Liver mu point, and the Gall Bladder mu point each lies on its own meridian, but the Kidney mu point lies on the Gall Bladder meridian, the Spleen mu point on the

Liver meridian, and the Large Intestine mu point on the Stomach meridian. Both the mu and the shu points may be used diagnostically – if they become tender or painful, this indicates a disturbance involving their associated meridian.

The choice of points to be used in treatment is therefore very complicated. The acupuncturist must know the function of each of the points on each of the meridians, along with the non-meridian extra points. She must know how the meridians interact with each other. She must know how to eliminate invasive conditions, such as cold and heat, from the body. She must know how to restore balance to the system and how to stimulate it to function normally once more. And, ideally, she must be able to do this while using a minimum of needles.

People are often worried at the thought of being stuck full of needles. But one of the skills of an expert acupuncturist lies in knowing how to treat a condition using the fewest possible acupuncture points. Often a patient may be treated with no more than four or five needles, and sometimes just a single needle will be enough. Five correctly chosen points will produce results just as effectively as ten. In the next chapter, a variety of illnesses is discussed, and a number of points are listed that might be used in the treatment of each of them. In some cases there may be a large number of suitable points, but it's important to remember that these would not all be used at the same time. However, where there is a wide range of equally appropriate points and where the treatment is carried out over a period of weeks or months, the practitioner might use all of them in rotation.

Although needling is probably the easiest, most effective, and therefore most popular way of stimulating the acupuncture points, treatment it is not always necessary to use a needle. Methods, which stimulate the points in other ways, are widely used, both to complement acupuncture and as an alternative in cases where the use of needles is inappropriate (for example, in the treatment of young children).

Acupressure

Acupressure is the treatment of the acupuncture points by massage. Usually the pressure is pulsed – in other words, applied and released a number of times. How long pressure is applied each time may depend on whether the point is tender. If it is, the therapist may press for only a second or two before resting. However, the patient will soon realise that, as treatment continues, the point becomes less tender. After a few uncomfortable minutes, he will be able to withstand pressure applied to the point for longer and longer periods. Since a tender acupuncture point is an indication that the point needs treating, the diminution of the tenderness shows that the treatment is working. This can be very encouraging to both patient and therapist.

There are, however, three drawbacks to acupressure. Firstly, only one point can be treated at a time (bilaterally if necessary), whereas more may be needed, particularly in patients with long-term problems. Secondly, the therapist must remain with the patient throughout the treatment, unlike acupuncture where, once the needles are in, the patient can be left alone for a few minutes while they take effect. Thirdly, the therapist needs to have very strong and resilient hands or he may find that he needs treatment himself – for painful thumbs!

Moxibustion

I mentioned in chapter 1 that moxibustion can be useful in the treatment of conditions that tend to be more prevalent in a damp climate. Moxa is still used today to treat conditions caused by cold and damp and, as you might expect, is especially useful in areas such as Japan, Great Britain, and the Pacific Northwest, where the climate tends to be damp much of the time. Certain points are particularly susceptible to treatment with moxa.

The usual method of using moxa is to attach a small wad of it to the end of an acupuncture needle that has been inserted into the relevant point. The moxa is lit, and the warmth it produces travels down the needle and into the point. Since the shortest needle in common use is an inch long and has a handle that is also an inch or more long, the moxa is never less than about an inch and a half away from the skin, so the patient is unlikely to get scorched.

Cupping

Cupping is another method of treating points that need warming in order to eliminate cold or damp. However, unlike moxibustion – which is applied to an individual point and can be used on any part of the body – cupping can only be used where there are large flat surfaces which are wide enough to take the cups, such as the back or the thighs. The cups, which are made of glass or bamboo, are heated, usually by inserting a burning taper inside them, which creates a partial vacuum. The taper is removed and the cup is immediately placed onto the skin, where it adheres via the suction created by the vacuum.

The cups are left on the skin for a few minutes before they are gently prised off, often leaving raised pink marks which usually disappear fairly rapidly. The suction produced by the cups is quite strong (this is what causes the pink marks, since blood is drawn into the surface vessels of the skin) – strong enough, it is said, to draw out the cold or damp causing the disease. Cupping is therefore very useful for conditions such as bronchitis where the acupuncturist has diagnosed an invasion by cold or damp and where the area affected – in this case the skin overlying the lung – can be covered using four to six cups. It is also considered effective in moving obstructions, and so may be used to treat patients in whom a blockage in the circulation of *qi* or of blood has been diagnosed.

Before we leave the subject of cupping, I need to mention its effect on sebaceous cysts. I've heard it said that the suction produced by cupping can be strong enough to cause a sebaceous cyst to burst, drawing out all the cheesy matter contained in it. However, although this may sound like a good way to eliminate a cyst, it actually isn't because the result will only be temporary. The cheesy matter making up a cyst is contained within a capsule and, unless this capsule is removed, the cyst will re-form. Since cupping is unable to remove the capsule (this has to be done surgically), the cyst is bound to recur. Not only this, but the breaking of the capsule (whether by cupping or by other means) can cause inflammation which can result in the capsule sticking to the surrounding tissues and so make its removal by surgery more difficult. If you have a sebaceous cyst, therefore, and you suspect that your acupuncturist is going to use cupping, ask her to avoid putting a cup over the cyst itself. Of course, the improved balance of the body's energies that results from treatment with acupuncture may result in a cyst gradually disappearing and should certainly help to prevent any new cysts from forming.

USE OF NEEDLES

Despite these various ways of stimulating acupuncture points, the most common form of treatment – and the one that everyone has heard of – is the insertion of needles into the points.

When people who are not familiar with acupuncture therapy hear about needles being stuck into patients, they invariably think of hypodermic needles, injections and, consequently, pain. Because of this they are often unable to understand how acupuncture can so frequently be quite painless. But there are two main reasons why injections are painful, and neither applies to acupuncture.

Firstly, because a fluid has to be passed down a hypodermic needle, the needle is hollow. As it enters the skin, it cuts out a tiny section and pushes it deeper into the tissues, causing pain. Secondly, the fluid is subsequently injected into the tissues and, because there is no natural cavity there to receive it, it compresses the tissue cells and nerve endings. This, too, is painful. An acupuncture needle, on the other hand, is very fine, it is not hollow, and nothing is forced down it. Thus its insertion feels quite unlike an injection.

Acupuncture needles come in lengths ranging from one to three inches, and each has a handle that is another inch or two long. At first glance, they may look fairly alarming. However, a needle is rarely inserted to its full length. In areas where there is just a thin layer of flesh overlying a bone, such as the forehead or the hands, only the tip of the needle is inserted. Deep insertion is only used in areas of thick muscle, such as the buttocks and the thighs.

The length of time that a needle is left in depends on the practitioner and on the treatment being given. Sometimes it is only appropriate to leave a needle in for a second or two. It may be that the purpose is just to puncture the skin and draw off a drop of blood, creating a passageway through which the body can rid itself of invasive *qi*. One practitioner I knew, who also practised manipulation, often inserted a needle briefly into a few points around the area that he intended to manipulate. This had the effect of loosening the surrounding muscles, making the manipulation easier and therefore more comfortable for the patient.

Some practitioners will attach needles to a machine that stimulates them with a mild electrical impulse, causing them to vibrate slightly and producing a mild buzzing sensation. With or without this stimulation, needles may be left in for a period of ten minutes or more. Once they have been inserted, however, the patient usually feels relaxed and comfortable and doesn't find the treatment in any way unpleasant. In fact, in the hands of an expert, patients have been known to feel so relaxed that they have dozed off.

Different techniques may be used to insert and remove the needles, according to whether the aim of the treatment is to stimulate the flow of *qi* (in a case of deficiency) or to sedate it (in a case of excess). In the former example, the acupuncturist might ask the patient to breathe out as she inserts the needle and to breathe in as she takes it out. Having extracted it, she may then massage the acupuncture point into which it was inserted.

With a patient who has an excess of *qi*, the needle might be inserted on an inhalation and removed on an exhalation, and might also be rotated while in place. A needle whose function is to stimulate *qi* may be inserted so that it lies in the direction of flow of *qi* along the meridian, while one intended to reduce *qi* might face in the opposite direction.

EAR ACUPUNCTURE

Some needles are designed to remain in position semi-permanently. These are the ear studs that are commonly used to help patients who wish to stop smoking or to lose weight. The method was developed in France in the mid-twentieth century by Paul Nogier who is often referred to as the father of modern ear acupuncture. It has become very popular, particularly with smokers who are desperate to quit. It is based on the idea that the human body is reflected, in microcosm, in three parts of itself – the hand, the foot and the ear. Any part of the body can therefore be treated through the corresponding part of the hand, foot or ear. (This is also the basis of another complementary therapy, reflexology, in which the therapist looks for areas of tenderness in the patient's feet or hands in order to identify problems in various parts of the body, and then treats them by massaging the appropriate points.)

In acupuncture, the ear is used in preference to the hand or the foot, but the principle is much the same. A tender area anywhere on the body suggests that the point needs to be treated. In the ear, it also implies an underlying disorder in the part of the body associated with that point. Ear acupuncture is especially useful in the treatment of small children or of patients who are squeamish about needles – inserting a single needle in a place where they cannot see it (and possibly hardly feel it) will cause minimum of distress. It is also valuable in the treatment of simple conditions where there is no long-standing disruption of *qi* involved. So, for a patient who has, say, a sprained ankle, inserting a single needle into the ear's ankle point may be an appropriate form of treatment.

When using the ear for the treatment of physical disorders, there is no need to leave the needles in for very long. However, patients who are trying to give up smoking or to diet need continuous help. For them, studs are used that can be left in for about two weeks at a time. These studs are made from a twist of stainless steel and look very much like tiny drawing pins. If a smoker is being treated, a stud is inserted into the lung point in the ear. For a dieter, a point in the centre of the area related to the digestive tract is used. The stud is held in by a small piece of adhesive tape. Inserting a stud may be slightly painful, since the ear is not a very fleshy area, but this pain should only be temporary and the patient should be perfectly comfortable within an hour or so. Because they are held in by tape, ear studs are not suitable for patients who are allergic to the adhesive. Nor are they suitable for those few patients who develop dermatitis when in prolonged contact with metal. I have heard of allergic patients, however, who were so desperate to give up smoking that they took a course of antihistamine tablets for the period of time that they needed the stud! A better way to do this, perhaps, would be to undergo a course of acupuncture to help resolve the allergies before going on to have an ear stud inserted.

Studs are a form of self-help. Every time the patient has a craving for a cigarette (or, in the case of a dieter, something to eat), she gently massages the stud with her finger for about ten or twenty seconds until the craving disappears. Western medicine, which likes to find an empirical reason for everything, has discovered that massaging the stud causes the body to release substances known as endorphins into the bloodstream. These naturally-occurring painkillers have an effect not dissimilar to that of morphine (hence the name). They probably do play a role in the action of the stud, but their release is unlikely to be the whole story. It doesn't explain why studs will only work if they are in exactly the right place, nor why a stud in the lung point won't help a dieter or why one in the digestive tract area won't help a smoker.

Of course, a stud will only reduce the physical craving or hunger pangs experienced by the patient. A mental desire to smoke or to eat cannot be inhibited by a stud, so the patient must really want to give up smoking or to lose weight. It may sound as though it is just a question of mind over matter. Still, there is no doubt that some patients find acupuncture studs work even when they have had no success with plain willpower or with other treatments – including hypnotherapy which is, unquestionably, a mind-over-matter treatment.

The great advantage of acupuncture studs is that they have no side effects. Unlike nicotine patches and appetite suppressants, no drug is entering the patient's system, so studs can continue to be used for as long as it takes the patient to achieve his goal. I knew one woman, who had a great deal of weight to lose, who used a stud for more than eighteen months, during which time she lost a steady two to three pounds a week – something she'd never been able to do before.

Although the treatment is perfectly safe for long-term use, the stud itself must be changed about every two weeks. This is because, even though the studs are sterile and made of stainless steel, if they stay in over longer periods of time they may act as a focus for infection. To avoid this risk, studs must be changed regularly. The ear used is alternated to reduce the risk still more. Patients are warned that if the stud becomes painful at any time, they should take it out. This is done simply by removing the adhesive tape, which will cause the stud to fall out. The ease with which studs can come out is important to remember when you wash your hair, take a shower, or if you go swimming, with a stud in your ear.

7

HOW ACUPUNCTURE WORKS: CASE HISTORIES

To those people who are used to the Western tradition of medicine, the Chinese diagnosis of illness in terms of invasion of the body by wind, heat, or other factors may seem bizarre. You must remember, however, that this method of diagnosis is many centuries old and, while practitioners may originally have believed that these invasions were taking place, it can be thought of nowadays as a kind of medical shorthand which indicates the form that the treatment should take. When an acupuncturist puts a needle into a point that is specific for dispelling wind from the body, he doesn't expect a rush of air to occur, as though it was being released from a pricked balloon. What he does expect, however, is that when he has diagnosed a disease as being due to invasion by wind, the use of such wind-dispelling points will enable him to improve the patient's condition.

In Western medicine, a single diagnosis does not necessarily mean that only one form of treatment is available to the patient. For example, a patient suffering from depression may be offered antidepressant tablets or psychotherapy – or both. A patient with cancer may be treated by surgery, radiotherapy or chemotherapy, or any combination of these. And if a condition is treated with medication, the doctor may be able to choose from among a large number of drugs that work in different ways. But in acupuncture, treatment is far more clear-cut. If a patient has a disease that has been caused by invasion by heat, then the treatment is to rid him of the excessive heat, to balance out any consequent imbalance of *yin* and *yang*, and to restore the flow of *qi* to normal.

For a patient in whom an injury has caused a blockage to the normal flow of *qi* (for example, a patient with a sprained ankle) and where pain is being caused by the blockage or by stagnant blood, the treatment is to release the block or disperse the blood. Naturally, this all sounds very unscientific, as well it might when you remember that these are the descriptions that have been in use for more than two thousand years. However, it is the indication that these descriptions give us as to treatment that is important. And since, in the hands of an expert, a diagnosis – and the treatment that automatically follows from it – can produce remarkably beneficial results, it seems unimportant that the diagnosis is couched in terms that have no relevance to modern Western medicine.

In this chapter, I want to look at some disorders that are commonly seen in Western medical practice and to consider how an acupuncturist might diagnose and treat them. In each case, points will be listed that the acupuncturist might use. However, it is important to note that these are not the only points that might be used and that, of those that are suitable, it is unlikely that more than four or five would be used at any one time. In addition, keep in mind that the exact location of the points will vary slightly from individual to individual. The unit of measurement used to locate acupuncture points is known as a cun (or, sometimes, a li) and, being based on bodily proportions, differs from person to person. For example, the breadth of the four fingers held lightly together is 3 cun, while the length of the forearm between the anterior elbow crease and the wrist crease is 12 cun.

Since in real life things are seldom as simple as they seem to be in textbooks, I will also include, at the end, some real case histories in which the points mentioned are those that were actually used by the practitioner.

ARTHRITIS

Since acupuncture is usually associated in people's minds with the idea of pain relief, arthritis is probably one of the most common complaints for which patients initially see an acupuncturist

Western medicine classifies the majority of arthritis cases as either osteoarthritis or rheumatoid arthritis. Osteoarthritis is a disease that results from wear and tear, and so occurs more commonly in older patients. In younger people it usually develops in joints that have previously been damaged (for example, by a sports injury). It often affects the large joints, particularly the hips, which have spent a lifetime carrying the body around. After a joint's natural surfaces have been worn away, deposits of calcium are laid down in it and the patient finds that the joint becomes stiff and causes pain, especially upon movement.

Rheumatoid arthritis, on the other hand, is an inflammatory condition that can affect people of any age, including children. On the whole, it attacks the smaller joints, which become inflamed and distorted. Some patients recover completely, whereas others may be left crippled. However, the majority of people who suffer from rheumatoid arthritis experience a certain degree of disability without it ever becoming severe. For some reason, this condition is much more common in women than in men.

The main feature of both types of arthritis is that the joints are painful and stiff and may be swollen. Chinese diagnosis ascribes these symptoms to a blockage in the flow of qi, either because the meridians affected have been invaded by external harmful *qi* or because a meridian has been damaged by injury.

Damage to a meridian may, at first, remain quite localised but, if it is untreated, the disruption to the flow of *qi* may spread and affect other meridians. For example, if a soccer player is kicked on the side of his knee, the area may become bruised and swollen but then resolve, so that the knee returns to normal. On the other hand, if he tries to play soccer while the joint is still recovering, this could interfere with healing and the condition could become chronic. A Western physician would say that the initial blow has set up a reaction within the joint and that, aggravated by further stress, this has resulted in the development of an arthritic condition. A Chinese physician might say that the initial blow disrupted the flow of *qi* in the Gall Bladder meridian, which runs down the side of the knee, and because the flow was not allowed to return to normal, the disruption has spread to involve the Urinary Bladder meridian (running down the back of the leg), the Stomach meridian (running down the front of the leg) and then the Liver, Kidney and Spleen meridians. Ultimately a circle formed around the knee through which the flow of *qi* was blocked.

It is the blockage of *qi* that causes the pain and the swelling. The acupuncturist's treatment will attempt to relieve the block and disperse any invasive *qi* that may have been the precipitating cause. However, arthritis often occurs in more than just one joint, and our athlete is not the typical arthritic patient.

Let us take the imaginary case of a middle-aged woman who comes to see the acupuncturist complaining of pain in her joints. She has had this for some years and it has gradually been getting worse. It is particularly bad if the weather is wet or cold but, to some extent, it is relieved by warmth – she finds that she is more mobile in the summer months. The pain in her wrists and the numbness and pain in her fingers make it increasingly difficult for her to do housework, sew or write out a shopping list.

Two important points in this history are that the condition is chronic (that is, long-term) and that it is made worse by cold and damp. It would seem, therefore, that cold and damp may be the external factors involved (since both of these tend to produce chronic conditions). Conditions that present with painful joints (including those that, in the West, are diagnosed as arthritis, rheumatic fever and gout) are commonly known in Chinese medicine as bi syndromes. Bi implies an obstruction – both to the flow of *qi* and to the blood. This woman would seem to have a bi syndrome resulting from an invasion by cold and damp.

On examination, this patient is found to have some swelling around the affected joints. This, too, suggests an obstruction to the flow of qi. Her tongue has a thin, moist, white coating – which, in a patient who is unwell, suggests an invasion by cold and damp. Finally, her pulse is deep and slow. This indicates that the condition is internal – and therefore chronic – and cold in nature.

To treat this patient, the acupuncturist would use points that disperse the invading cold and damp and remove the obstruction to the flow of qi. Because of the chronicity of the condition, the body's production of protective *qi* also needs to be stimulated, to help the patient to fight back. And the acupuncturist might also treat specific areas, such as the wrists and hands, that are particularly troublesome. Table 1 shows some of the points that might be used.

TABLE 1: TREATMENT OF A PATIENT WITH OSTEOARTHRITIS

Moxibustion, with its effect of warming the acupuncture points, would be particularly useful in counteracting the invasive cold and damp. The overall effect of treatment will be to unblock obstructed meridians, clear out invading cold and damp, and stimulate the circulation of blood and *qi* around the body. Of course, it may happen that the patient's hands and wrists are too painful to withstand the insertion of needles on the first visit. In this case the acupuncturist will use the points located further away from the painful areas and will begin to use the local points only as the patient's condition improves.

Now let's look at a patient who, in Western terms, has had an acute attack of rheumatoid arthritis. The interesting thing here is that both this patient and the middle-aged woman just described might be treated by a Western practitioner with the same sorts of drugs – painkillers, anti-inflammatory preparations and, possibly, even steroids. To an acupuncturist, however, the two patients are treated quite differently from each other because they are diagnosed as suffering from different conditions.

Let us assume that this second patient is a thirty year old woman who has recently developed swelling and pain in several of her joints. She has a mild fever and the affected joints are red and feel hot to the touch. Unlike the older woman, her pain is not constant. Some days her knees are the most painful, on other days it is her wrists, and sometimes her feet are the most troublesome.

Listening to her story, the acupuncturist decides that there has been an invasion by heat (causing the redness of the joints and the fever) and by wind (causing the pain to flit from one joint to another). Looking at her, he sees that her face is flushed, indicating the presence of a hot disease. Her tongue is red and has a yellow coating and her pulse is rapid and forceful, all of which confirms the diagnosis of an invasion by heat.

Some of the points the acupuncturist might use to treat rheumatoid arthritis are shown in table 2. Here again, the overall effect of treatment is to dispel the causative factors – in this case, wind and heat – and to unblock obstructions to the flow of qi. Once *qi* is flowing normally again and the heat and wind have been dispersed, the patient's joints will be able to return to normal.

TABLE 2: TREATMENT OF A PATIENT WITH RHEUMATOID ARTHRITIS

Point	Name	Meaning	Location	Action
LI 11	Quchi	Crooked pool	In a depression at the lateral side of the elbow crease	Eliminates heat and wind; used for its local effects on the wrist; reduces pain and swelling in joints
LI 15	Jianyu	Corner of shoulder	Just below the point of the shoulder	Eliminates heat and wind; eliminates stagnant *qi*; specific for pain in the shoulder joint
St 45	Lidui	Door of the stomach	At the end of the meridian, on the second toe, just behind the corner of the nail	Eliminates wind; has a specific action on the knees and feet
UB 12	Fengmen	Gate of the wind	To the side of the spine, approximately level with the upper point of the shoulder blade, at a point where the body is easily invaded by wind	Specific for arthritic conditions, particularly when caused by wind
SJ 5	Waiguan	Lateral pass	Just above the wrist, on the lateral side of the humerus	Eliminates heat; local point for treating the wrist

MIGRAINE

This is another complaint that often finds its way into the acupuncturist's clinic, since Western medicine cannot always treat it successfully.

Although migraine still isn't fully understood, it is believed usually to be triggered by factors such as stress, over-tiredness or female hormone fluctuations. This causes nerve cells in the brain to become over-excited. They fire off impulses erratically and this causes the early symptoms such as nausea and flashing lights. After this, it seems that levels of the neurotransmitter serotonin drop and this causes the blood vessels in the brain to dilate, producing the headache. Once the migraine has developed, ordinary painkillers such as aspirin and paracetamol usually have little effect on it. The aim of Western medical treatment is to stop the migraine before it gets to this stage by preventing the arteries from behaving in this abnormal way. The ergot derivatives that form the basis of a number of migraine treatments are vasoconstrictors – in other words, they prevent overdilation of the arteries and so stop the headache from developing.

Let us now look at a young woman who comes to the acupuncture clinic complaining of recurrent migraine. She describes the pain that she experiences during an attack as running from just above one eye across the top of her head and down into her neck. It is severe and throbbing, and her face becomes hot and flushed.

And let us say that, on the way to her appointment, the patient starts to develop a migraine. By the time she sees the acupuncturist, the headache is becoming quite severe. Looking at her, the acupuncturist sees that her face is red, indicating a hot condition. When he examines her eyes, they appear inflamed, and she complains that the light hurts them. This suggests that the heat is a result of an excess of *yang*. Her tongue is red and has a yellow coating, which again signifies heat. Her pulse is rapid due to the heat, and is both forceful and floating in character, indicating an external syndrome with an excess of *yang*.

The treatment of this patient, therefore, would be aimed at reducing this overabundance of *yang* and bringing *yin* and *yang* back into balance. This will then cool the heat that has arisen as a result of excessive *yang*. The path that the pain takes – from the eye, across the head, and into the neck – corresponds to the route of the Gall Bladder meridian in this part of the body, a meridian that is often out of balance in patients with migraine. The acupuncturist may feel along the course of the meridian for tender points that need treatment. One acupuncture teacher I knew called them, rather accurately, 'ouch points', but their Chinese name is *ah-shi* (meaning 'oh, yes!') points. If the patient has been suffering from recurrent migraine, these points will probably be tender even between attacks.

Treatment can either be given during the migraine itself, to stop the attack, or between migraines when the patient feels well. In either case, the balancing out of *yin* and *yang* should help to prevent further attacks. The patient may also be advised to stop smoking, drinking alcohol, and eating red meat, since these are factors that can stimulate the formation of excess *yang*.

Table 3 shows some of the points that might be used in the treatment of this patient.

TABLE 3: TREATMENT OF A PATIENT WITH MIGRAINE

Point	Name	Meaning	Location	Action
St 8	Touwei	Corner of the head	At the corner of the forehead, just within the hairline	A specific point for the treatment of migraine
SJ 5	Waiguan	Lateral pass	Just above the wrist on the lateral side of the humerus	An important point for treating external conditions, clearing heat and restoring *yang* to normal
GB 14	Yangbai	*Yang* brightness	A little way above the midpoint of the eyebrow	May be an *ah-shi* point in this condition; brightens the eyes (hence the name)
GB 17	Zheng-ying	Fright and fear	Just lateral to the crown of the head	May be an *ah-shi* point in this condition; can treat fright and fear (hence the name)
GB 20	Fengchi	Wind pool	At the back of the neck, in the depression below the base of the skull	May be an *ah-shi* point in this condition; an important point for eliminating wind
GB 41	Zulinqui	Foot treating tears	On the lateral side of the foot	Indicated in the treatment of a number of eye conditions

ASTHMA AND BRONCHITIS

These two conditions can be either acute or chronic, and they can affect people of any age. Western medicine has little to offer in the way of cure once they have become chronic, although it can often control them very effectively through the use of drugs. However, many people do not like the idea of having to take drugs for the rest of their lives, and some start to look for an alternative form of therapy.

During an asthma attack, the bronchi, or tubes, in the lungs constrict and so impede the flow of air into and out of the lungs. The condition is becoming increasingly prevalent, especially in young people. In many cases, it is caused by an allergy – often to pollen, so that an attack of hay fever may lead into an attack of asthma. In other cases, children who have had eczema (another allergic condition) sometimes develop asthma later on, although their skin condition may improve. This would be an indication to an acupuncturist that the disease was turning from an external syndrome into an internal one. Treatment might well result in a return of the eczema before the patient's recovery is complete.

In many cases of allergic asthma, the allergen (the substance to which the patient is allergic) is house dust. Other common allergens are feathers and animal fur, so birds, cats, dogs and horses will set off an attack if they come near the patient. Asthma also has a psychological component – it can be a very frightening condition, and the fear that arises when an attack starts may itself make the attack worse, forming a vicious circle.

Asthma may be associated with bronchitis in an individual patient, but the two conditions can occur independently of each other. Bronchitis is an inflammatory condition of the bronchi brought on by anything that causes the lungs to become inflamed, such as infection or smoking. An acute attack, which presents as a bad cough accompanied by the production of large amounts of yellow or green phlegm, and which is due to a bacterial infection, may be completely cured by treatment with antibiotics. However, a series of attacks can cause permanent damage to the lungs. This is especially likely to happen if the attacks are inadequately treated, if there is another contributory condition such as asthma present, or if the patient is a smoker, which will prevent the bronchitis from ever resolving completely. If this is the case, the patient may go on to develop chronic bronchitis, with a permanent productive cough and shortness of breath – a condition commonly seen in patients who have smoked heavily for years.

Let us take as an example, first of all, a patient who would be diagnosed by a Western physician as having asthma. He is a young man who periodically develops a tight feeling in his chest that makes it difficult for him to breathe. During these attacks, which can be brought on if he gets stressed or overtired, he wheezes and coughs up some white frothy sputum. On examination, he is found to have a sticky white coating on his tongue and a slow pulse that feels like a taut wire. From these symptoms and signs, the acupuncturist can diagnose that the patient has congestion in his lungs attributable to invasion by cold (because the pulse is slow) and by phlegm (because of the sputum and the appearance of the tongue). The bowstring pulse indicates that the congestion is secondary to spasm, which is preventing the normal flow of qi. This type of asthma is also said to be brought on by exposure to a cold wind when the patient is tired, and it may be made worse by emotion.

Treatment of this patient by a Western physician would use drugs to relax the spasms in the bronchi. An acupuncturist, on the other hand, would select points to disperse the cold and the phlegm, and use moxa or cupping to warm the lungs. Some of the points that might be used are shown in table 4.

TABLE 4: TREATMENT OF A PATIENT WITH COLD-INDUCED ASTHMA

Our second hypothetical patient is somewhat older than the first – in his fifties – but presents with the same tight feeling in his chest and wheezy breathing. In addition, he has a slight fever and a chesty cough. The spasms in his chest prevent him from coughing up very much sputum, but what does come up is thick and either yellow or green. On examination, his pulse is fast and slippery or gliding in quality. His tongue is red and has a sticky yellow coating. The diagnosis here is one of invasion of the lungs by heat, which has caused stagnation of *qi* and the formation of phlegm. This is indicated by the fever, fast pulse, and red tongue with yellow coating, all of which signify heat, while the slippery pulse, sputum and stickiness of the tongue coating all point to the presence of phlegm.

A Western doctor would prescribe a bronchorelaxant drug and an antibiotic. An acupuncturist could choose from among a number of points, some of which are shown in table 5.

TABLE 5: TREATMENT OF A PATIENT WITH HEAT-INDUCED ASTHMA

Point	Name	Meaning	Location	Action
Lu 5	Chize	Ulnar marsh	In a depression next to the ulna bone, in the crease of the elbow	Clears heat from the lung; alleviates stagnation; an important point for regulating the *qi* of the lung
St 40	Fenlong	Great abundance	On the lateral side of the leg, at the lowest part of the calf, at a point where *qi* flows abundantly	Eliminates phlegm
UB 13	Feishu	Lung *shu* point	To the side of the spine, near the upper border of the shoulder blade	Strengthens the *qi* of the lung and promotes its circulation; removes blockages in the lung
Ren 22	Tiantu	Chimney of heaven	In the midline depression at the base of the neck, above the breastbone, where the windpipe acts as a chimney for the *qi* of the lung	An important local point for the treatment of respiratory diseases and has a specific effect in the treatment of asthma; stimulates the circulation of *qi* in the lung

Still on the topic of asthma, let us finally look at a child who has chronic asthma and whom a Western physician would treat in a similar way to the two patients already mentioned. This little boy, let us say, is eight years old and has had asthma since the age of three. The recurrent attacks have interfered with his normal development, and he is underweight and short for his age. He gets tired easily and is inclined to be restless. On examination, his face has a yellowish tinge, and his lips are pale. His tongue, too, is pale and it has a thin, white, sticky coating. His pulse feels forceless and disappears on pressure. The characteristics of his pulse, along with the colour of his face and lips, suggest that this is a xu, or deficiency, condition. This is also suggested by his pale tongue and by the fact that he is small and underweight. The sticky white coating on his tongue points to an invasion by cold and damp or phlegm. The deficiency has obviously affected the lungs, producing the symptoms of asthma but, since the kidney is the organ in charge of growth and development, there would seem to be a deficiency there as well. According to the Law of the Five Elements, the Lung meridian, which is Metal, is mother to the Kidney meridian which is, of course, Water. So a long-term deficiency in one can easily affect the other.

One possible treatment for this patient is shown in table 6. Obviously, a long-term problem such as this would need an extended course of treatment. The points used would probably vary from session to session, too, depending on how the condition was reacting.

TABLE 6: TREATMENT OF A CHILD WITH CHRONIC ASTHMA

Point	Name	Meaning	Location	Action
Lu 9	Taiyuan	Great abundant pool	On the wrist above the thumb, at a point where the *qi* of the meridian is abundant	Eliminates phlegm; forms a direct link with the lung and can be used to stimulate it; as Earth point of the Lung meridian, it can be used in accordance with the Law of the Five Elements *
UB 13	Feishu	Lung *shu* point	To the side of the spine, near the upper border of the shoulder blade	Removes blockages in the lung; strengthens the *qi* of the lung and stimulates its circulation
UB 23	Shenshu	Kidney *shu* point	To the side of the spine, at about the level of the waist	Stimulates the functional *qi* of the kidney
K 3	Taixi	Great canyon	On the medial aspect of the ankle, in the depression beside the Achilles tendon	Stimulates the functional *qi* of the kidney
Du 4	Mingmen	Door of life	Along the midline of the back, at the level of the kidney, whose *qi* is the basic source for the whole body	Stimulates the functional *qi* of the kidney

**The Lung, which is the yin Metal meridian, is the child of the Spleen, the yin Earth meridian. Lu 9 is the Earth point of the Lung meridian and so can be used to stimulate the mother (the Spleen meridian) to nourish her child. (See chapter 3)*

Of course, as I have already noted, asthma and bronchitis can exist independently of each other and so, to round off this section, let us bring into our imaginary acupuncture clinic two patients suffering from bronchitis – one with the acute condition, the other with the chronic.

Let us say that the first of these patients became ill a week or so ago when he developed a head cold with a runny nose, fever, and general feeling of being unwell. Since then, he has started to cough and is bringing up quantities of thick, yellow sputum. Such complaints are, of course, regularly seen in general practitioners' surgeries during the winter months, and they are usually treated with a course of antibiotics. On examining the patient, the acupuncturist finds that he has a rapid pulse, a flushed face, and a red tongue with a thin yellow coating. All these factors point to a diagnosis of an invasion by heat. The thin yellow coating on the tongue suggests that wind may also be involved. If wind invades the lungs and blocks the circulation of qi, phlegm will form, and the fact that the patient has been coughing up sputum is another indication that this is what has happened. Table 7 shows some of the points that might be used to treat this patient.

TABLE 7: TREATMENT OF A PATIENT WITH ACUTE BRONCHITIS

The treatment of the patient with chronic bronchitis is somewhat different. He complains of a constant cough that becomes worse in winter, along with a lack of appetite and energy. Western medicine applies the term bronchitis to him as well as to the last patient because both are seen as having an inflammation ('-itis') of the tubes of the lungs (bronchi). However, Chinese medicine always emphasises the fundamental difference between acute and chronic conditions. Acute implies external and often hot syndromes, possibly with an excess of *yang*, while chronic suggests internal, cold and excessively *yin* syndromes.

TABLE 8: TREATMENT OF A PATIENT WITH CHRONIC BRONCHITIS

Point	Name	Meaning	Location	Action
Lu 9	Taiyuan	Great abundant pool	On the wrist above the thumb, at a point where the *qi* of the meridian is abundant	Eliminates phlegm; forms a direct link with the lung and can be used to stimulate it; stimulates the Earth meridians, encouraging the Spleen meridian to nourish its child, the Lung meridian*
UB 20	Pishu	Spleen *shu* point	To the side of the spine, above the level of the waist and below the shoulder blade	Acts in the same way as Lu 9*; promotes the circulation of *qi*
UB 23	Shenshu	Kidney *shu* point	To the side of the spine, at about the level of the waist	Stimulates the kidney to prevent any deficiency in that meridian from contributing to the deficiency of the lung^
K 3	Taixi	Great canyon	On the medial aspect of the ankle, in the depression beside the Achilles tendon	Acts in the same way as UB 23^

**The spleen is responsible for the transport and transformation of the nutrients that form qi. If it malfunctions, retention of water in the body can result. This may materialise in the lung as phlegm.*

^Because the Kidney meridian is the yin Water meridian and therefore the child of the Lung meridian, UB 23 and K 3 are used to stimulate the kidney. (See chapter 3.)

When the acupuncturist examines the chronic bronchitic patient, he finds a pale tongue and a deep, slow pulse. These, together with his symptoms of poor appetite and little energy, suggest a *xu* (deficiency) syndrome. The patient's tongue has a sticky, white coating, which indicates that cold and damp or phlegm are factors in the causation of the disease. So treatment would be aimed at stimulating the energy of the lungs and eliminating the cold and phlegm.

Table 8 shows the points that might be used to treat this patient. Naturally, a patient with chronic bronchitis will need a much longer course of treatment than one with acute bronchitis in order to obtain relief from his symptoms.

GALLBLADDER DISEASE

This is not a problem that you might immediately think of taking to an acupuncturist for treatment, since in Western practice it is usually dealt with surgically. Western physicians divide it into two main types: cholecystitis (inflammation of the gallbladder) and cholelithiasis (gallstones). Very often the two occur together. Both are painful conditions and commonly occur in women around the age of forty; the patients are frequently overweight.

Cholecystitis often has an acute onset, with the patient complaining of a constant, severe pain just under the base of the rib cage on the right-hand side, sometimes accompanied by fever and vomiting. Usually the cause is an infection, sometimes due to the fact that there are stones in the galllader, and Western treatment might consist of antibiotics in the acute stage followed by removal of the gallbladder later on when the infection has settled down.

When uncomplicated by infection, gallstones are more likely to be associated with a colicky, or spasmodic, pain due to the gallbladder trying to squeeze the stone out, or to a stone actually passing down the bile duct leading from the gallbladder to the small intestine. In either condition, jaundice may occur if the flow of bile into the small intestine is blocked either by the inflammation or by a stone. Because the symptoms of the two complaints can be very similar, it may be necessary to take Xrays to establish whether or not gallstones are present. A gallbladder that contains stones is usually removed together with the stones.

In order to see how such a patient might be treated by acupuncture, let us imagine that an acupuncturist is called to see a thirty nine year old woman who is complaining of severe pain under the right side of her rib cage, along with fever and jaundice. On examination, her tongue is found to be red with a sticky yellow coating, and her pulse is rapid and forceful. The location of the pain indicates a problem with the liver and gallbladder, which lie together under the right-hand border of the rib cage. Jaundice is usually seen as an indication of invasion by damp heat. This is corroborated by the appearance of the patient's tongue and her fever. The forceful quality of her pulse suggests a *shi* (excess) syndrome, and the involvement of heat further suggests that it is *yang* that is in excess.

Some points that the acupuncturist might use are shown in table 9. It is important to remember that no therapy can be 100 per cent successful every time and that, sometimes, the best results are achieved by a combination of two therapies. Gallbladder disease may be a case in point, with acupuncture being used to treat the acute attack, followed by surgery to remove the offending organ and its stones.

TABLE 9: TREATMENT OF A PATIENT WITH GALLBLADDER DISEASE

Point	Name	Meaning	Location	Action
UB 18	Ganshu	Liver *shu* point	Lateral to the spine, between the armpit and the waist	Stimulates *qi*, relieves obstruction
UB 19	Danshu	Gall Bladder *shu* point	Just below UB 18	Stimulates *qi*, relieves obstruction
GB 34	Yangling-quan	*Yang* mound spring	In a depression below the bony prominence on the lateral aspect of the knee	Stimulates *qi*, relieves obstruction
Liv 2	Xingjian	Walking in the middle	Between the first and second toes	Reduces heat in the liver, mobilises *qi* that has become stuck*
Liv 3	Taichong	Great pass	On the upper aspect of the foot, along a line that runs between the first and second toes	Reduces heat; suppresses excess *yang*
Ren 12	Zhong-wan	Middle of stomach	Along the midline of the abdomen, a little way above the umbilicus	Expels damp heat

**Liv 2 is also the Fire point of the meridian. Fire is the child of Wood, and the Liver and Gall Bladder are both Wood meridians. In a shi syndrome, it is customary to treat the child while, in a xu syndrome, the mother is the one that is treated. (See chapter 3.)*

HYPERTENSION (HIGH BLOOD PRESSURE)

Although modern drugs can control hypertension very effectively in the majority of cases, they may cause side effects. In addition, it is usually necessary for the patient to continue to take the tablets for the rest of his life. A therapy such as acupuncture, which does not have these drawbacks, may therefore seem more attractive.

In the West, hypertension is categorised as either primary or secondary. Secondary hypertension, as its name suggests, occurs as a result of another medical condition such as kidney disease or thyroid disease or may be a side effect of certain medications. Primary hypertension (also known as essential hypertension) is less clear cut but is more likely to occur in certain groups of people, such as those over 65, those who are obese, heavy drinkers, and those with a family history of the condition.

Hypertension often produces no symptoms in its early stages and is picked up only when the patient has his blood pressure checked during a routine medical examination. If undetected and therefore untreated, however, it may ultimately make itself known when the patient suffers a heart attack or a stroke.

As we have seen, diagnoses in Chinese medicine are based upon the patient's symptoms and outward signs, backed up by pulse and tongue observations. Elevated blood pressure per se is not recognised in traditional Chinese medicine because, naturally, when acupuncture was first used thousands of years ago, there was no equipment for measuring it. However, if a patient who has no symptoms but whose blood pressure has been found to be raised on testing goes to an acupuncturist, examination of his tongue and pulse (plus the other signs used by practitioners of the Five Elements school) should indicate a diagnosis in Chinese medical terms, and his treatment will be based on this.

Let us consider, for example, a patient who has already developed symptoms from her hypertension. She is a lady in her eighties, rather frail, who is complaining of slight dizziness, blurred vision, and recurring headaches. She also has difficulty sleeping and wakes early in the morning. Her face is pale but she has pink cheeks. Her tongue is red and slightly glossy in appearance, and she has a weak and rapid pulse.

Hypertension can be due either to an excess of *yang* or an excess of phlegm and damp. In this woman's case, the former would seem to be the cause. It is suggested by her pale face and pink cheeks, which indicate a *yin* deficiency resulting in a relative excess of *yang*. Such a deficiency may occur in the liver or kidney (which control the circulation of qi) simply as a result of growing old. A *yin* deficiency in the kidney will result in its child, the liver, becoming undernourished. The resulting relative hyperactivity of the liver's *yang* may produce dizziness. Headaches, a red tongue, and a rapid pulse also indicate an excess of *yang* (producing an inner heat), while a coexisting deficiency of *yin* is suggested by the blurred vision, sleeping problems, glossy tongue, and weakness of the pulse. Blurred vision is particularly associated with a deficiency in the liver, which is linked to the eye.

This patient may be helped by treatment using some of the points shown in table 10.

TABLE 10: TREATMENT OF A PATIENT WITH EXCESS YANG HYPERTENSION

Point	Name	Meaning	Location	Action
UB 23	Shenshu	Kidney *shu* point	To the side of the spine, at about the level of the waist	Stimulates the functional *qi* of the kidney
K 3	Taixi	Great canyon	On the medial aspect of the ankle, in the depression beside the Achilles tendon	Stimulates the *yin* and sedates the *yang* of the liver and kidney
Liv 2	Xingjian	Walking in the middle	Between the first and second toes	Stimulates *yin* and sedates *yang*; often used with Liv 3 in the control of hypertension
Liv 3	Taichong	Great pass	On the upper aspect of the foot, along a line that runs between the first and second toes	Reinforces the *yin* element of the kidney and liver; usually used with Liv 2 in the control of hypertension

If hypertension is caused by an invasion of phlegm and damp, the picture is quite different. We may imagine, in this case, a middle-aged man who, like the previous patient, complains of dizziness but, unlike her, is not frail but overweight. He also suffers from palpitations and occasional chest pain. On examination, he is found to have a slow and deep pulse, and his tongue has a sticky coating. Because it is related to eating habits, obesity is said to have a damaging effect on the spleen, which distills *qi* from ingested food. As a result, the formation and circulation of *qi* is affected. The sticky coating on this patient's tongue suggests that phlegm and damp have developed in conjunction with the poor circulation of qi. His deep, slow pulse indicates an internal syndrome and corroborates the findings on the tongue.

Retention of phlegm and damp within the body causes mental clouding and would be the reason for this patient's dizziness. His treatment consists of clearing out the phlegm and thus returning the function of the spleen to normal. Some of the points that might be used are shown in table 11.

TABLE 11: TREATMENT OF A PATIENT WITH PHLEGM- AND DAMP-INDUCED HYPERTENSION

Point	Name	Meaning	Location	Action
St 40	Fenglong	Great abundance	On the lateral aspect of the leg, at the lowest part of the calf, at a point where *qi* flows abundantly	Eliminates phlegm and damp
Liv 2	Xingjian	Walking in the middle	Between the first and second toes	Mobilises *qi* that has become obstructed
Ren 12	Zhong-wan	Middle of stomach	Along the midline of the abdomen, a little way above the umbilicus	Expels damp; a specific point for treating hypertension

URTICARIA

In Western medicine, urticaria (hives) is seen as an allergic problem and often occurs as a reaction to eating things such as shellfish or strawberries. It may also occur as a result of emotional trauma. Its other name is nettle rash, because the rash that it produces looks very similar to that which might be seen on someone who has been badly stung by nettles.

If we picture a woman with urticaria, she has large raised red patches on her arms, legs, trunk and face. These appeared suddenly and are hot and itchy. On examination, her tongue is red with a thin yellow coating, and her pulse is superficial in character and rapid. The redness of her skin patches, together with her red tongue and rapid pulse, suggest an invasion by heat, while the sudden onset and the yellow coating on the tongue indicate that wind is also involved. Treatment will therefore aim at eliminating both of these factors. Table 12 shows some of the points that might be used.

TABLE 12: TREATMENT OF A PATIENT WITH URTICARIA

Point	Name	Meaning	Location	Action
LI 4	Hegu	Valley junction	On the back of the hand, in the angle between the thumb and forefinger	Eliminates heat; is specific for the treatment of skin conditions
LI 11	Quchi	Crooked pool	In a depression at the lateral side of the elbow crease	Eliminates heat and wind
Sp 10	Xuehai	Sea of blood	On the inside of the leg, just above the bend of the knee	Eliminates heat; stimulates the flow of *qi*; is often used to treat inflamed skin conditions
UB 17	Geshu	Diaphragm *shu* point	To the side of the spine, at a point between the level of the armpit and that of the lower border of the shoulder blade	Eliminates wind by treating the blood and returning its flow to normal

TINNITUS (RINGING IN THE EARS)

This is another fairly common chronic problem but, unfortunately, one for which Western medicine doesn't have a lot to offer. It can be helped by various complementary therapies, however, including hypnotherapy, homoeopathy and, of course, acupuncture.

In Western medical terms, tinnitus is caused by damage to the nerve that supplies the inner ear; it is therefore usually associated with deafness. The patient's hearing is poor on two counts: firstly, due to the nerve damage and, secondly, because the tinnitus masks whatever sounds are able to get through. So, if the tinnitus can be diminished, the patient will hear better, whether or not the deafness itself has been reduced.

Let us take as our example a patient with what is known in Western terms as Ménière's disease (or Ménière's syndrome), which consists of ringing in the ears, dizziness, and gradually worsening deafness. He is a man in his seventies, and he tells the acupuncturist that his tinnitus becomes worse if he gets upset or stressed. He has a weak pulse, and his tongue looks pale.

TABLE 13: TREATMENT OF A PATIENT WITH TINNITUS

Point	Name	Meaning	Location	Action
Sp 6	Sanyin-jiao	Three *yin* meridians crossing	At the intersection point of the Spleen, Liver and Kidney meridians, on the medial aspect of the leg, a short way above the ankle	Stimulates the kidney and liver*
UB 23	Shenshu	Kidney *shu* point	To the side of the spine, at about the level of the waist	Stimulates the functional *qi* of the kidney
K 3	Taixi	Great canyon	On the medial aspect of the ankle, in the depression beside the Achilles tendon	Stimulates the functional *qi* of the kidney
GB 2	Tinghui	Gathering of hearing	Just in front of the ear, at the joint of the jaw	A specific point for treating deafness and tinnitus, due to its position next to the ear
Liv 3	Taichong	Great pass	On the upper aspect of the foot, along a line that runs between the first and second toes	Reinforces the *yin* element of the kidney and liver
Du 4	Mingmen	Door of life	Along the midline of the back, at the level of the kidney	Stimulates the functional *qi* of the kidney

**Here again, the treatment is based on the relationship between the Kidney (Water) meridian and the Liver (Wood) meridian. The former is the mother of the latter, and a deficiency in one will, if long continued, affect the other. (See chapter 3.)*

I noted above, in connection with the older lady with hypertension, that advanced age may be associated with reduced functioning of the kidney and a reduction in its functional qi. The sense organ with which the kidney is linked is the ear, so a chronic deficiency of *qi* in older people may reduce the ear's ability to function normally and thus cause deafness. This patient's deep, weak pulse and his pale tongue, together with the fact that his symptoms are aggravated by stress, all suggest the presence of a *xu* (deficiency) syndrome. The dizziness is due to a deficiency in the brain (or Sea of Marrow), whose maintenance is dependent on the normal functioning of the kidney.

In treatment, the aim is to strengthen the kidney and reinforce its functional qi. This may be done by using some of the points shown in table 13.

DEPRESSION

This is not the sort of problem you might, at first, think could be helped by acupuncture. We often tend to associate the use of acupuncture with purely physical problems, and even though there is no doubt that an imbalance of chemicals in the brain can cause clinical depression, it is primarily a mental condition. The truth, however, is that acupuncture can have remarkable effects on mental states. Like many other complementary therapies, it treats the whole patient by raising his entire level of health, thus increasing his ability to shake off whatever symptoms are troubling him, whether they be physical or mental.

Here we may imagine a middle-aged woman who is complaining of depression that has crept up on her very gradually over the past few months. She also feels very anxious, often without knowing why – a common accompaniment to depression. She has difficulty sleeping and experiences the early-morning wakefulness typical of clinical depression, waking at around five in the morning and being unable to fall asleep again. She also has occasional bouts of dizziness and feels totally devoid of energy all the time. On examination, her face is pale and her skin looks dull. Her tongue appears flabby, and there are indentations around its edge made by her teeth. Her pulse is slow and disappears upon pressure. These findings, together with her symptoms, all point to a deficiency syndrome. Since the heart is the seat of the mind, it would seem that her deficiency of *qi* has affected the Heart meridian. Treatment would therefore be aimed at stimulating the production and circulation of *qi* and ensuring adequate nourishment of the heart.

Table 14 shows some of the points that might be used for treating this woman.

TABLE 14: TREATMENT OF A PATIENT WITH DEPRESSION

Point	Name	Meaning	Location	Action
H 3	Shaohai	Young sea	At the medial end of the elbow crease, where the qi of the meridian circulates, like water flowing	An important point for the treatment of depression, strengthening the heart
H 7	Shenmen	Door of the mind	On the crease of the wrist, above the little finger	Strengthens the *qi* of the heart
UB 15	Xinshu	Heart *shu* point	To the side of the spine, a little above the level of the armpit	Strengthens the *qi* of the heart
UB 20	Pishu	Spleen *shu* point	To the side of the spine, above the level of the waist and below the shoulder blade	Stimulates the spleen; promotes the absorption and circulation of *qi**
UB 21	Weishu	Stomach *shu* point	To the side of the spine, above the level of the waist and just below UB 20	Stimulates the stomach; promotes the absorption and circulation of *qi**

**A general lowering of qi in the body may result from a malfunction of the spleen or stomach, which are responsible for extracting qi from ingested food.*

INSOMNIA

Many people suffer from insomnia at one time or another. Usually it is a temporary problem often caused by the patient going through a stressful period. If he is prepared to wait, he is likely to find that the problem resolves itself as soon as the stress has passed. However, many patients become so anxious about their inability to sleep that this anxiety itself contributes to the insomnia, turning an acute state into a chronic problem. While sleeping tablets may be a temporary solution, doctors nowadays tend to be unwilling to prescribe them for more than a few weeks for three reasons – firstly, they can become addictive; secondly, they tend to become less effective over time; and lastly, when the patient does come off them, he can find that the insomnia is now worse than it was before he started to take the medication.

Some acupuncturists believe that the effects of sleeping tablets and other tranquilisers on the system counteract the effects of acupuncture to some extent. So, if the patient is taking these, he may be asked to stop doing so before he starts treatment. However, other acupuncturists will treat a patient while he is still taking the tablets, allowing him to come off them in his own time, once the treatment starts to take effect.

Let us take as our example here a middle-aged man who has found it increasingly difficult to sleep over the past few months. When he does manage to fall asleep, he dreams a great deal. He says that, as a result of his sleeplessness, he gets dizzy, has an intermittent ringing in his ears, and is becoming very irritable. He is also getting pains in his back, which he attributes to his tossing and turning at night. His face is pale but his lips are red. His eyes look dull and his tongue is red and thin. His pulse is rapid and disappears on pressure.

From the fact that this condition is affecting the patient's mind (with sleeplessness, dreams, and irritability), we can determine that his heart – the seat of the mind – has been affected. The irritability, red lips, and rapid pulse are all indicative of heat. Still, his pale face and disappearing pulse speak of a deficiency. Dullness of the eyes suggests a deficiency of *yin* in the kidney. As we saw in the case of the older lady with hypertension, dizziness can be caused by hyperactivity of the liver's *yang*, secondary to inadequate nourishment of *yin* by the kidney. A thin red tongue is indicative of a deficiency of *yin* producing internal heat due to the relative excess of *yang*.

TABLE 15: TREATMENT OF A PATIENT WITH INSOMNIA

Point	Name	Meaning	Location	Action
H 7	Shenmen	Door of the mind	On the crease of the wrist, above the little finger	Strengthens the *qi* of the heart
UB 15	Xinshu	Heart *shu* point	To the side of the spine, a little above the level of the armpit	Strengthens the *qi* of the heart
UB 23	Sheshu	Kidney *shu* point	To the side of the spine, at about the level of the waist	Stimulates the functional *qi* of the kidney
K 3	Taixi	Great canyon	On the medial aspect of the ankle, in the depression beside the Achilles tendon	Stimulates the functional *qi* of the kidney; controls mental problems that have arisen as a result of a disharmony between the kidney and the heart

The meridian that has, so to speak, got out of control here is the Heart meridian. According to the servant-master relationship, the Heart meridian is the servant of the Kidney meridian, so a deficiency in the latter could produce symptoms of overactivity or heat in the former. Treatment should therefore stimulate the function of the kidney while sedating the activity of the heart.

Table 15 shows some of the points that might be used to achieve this.

BELL'S PALSY (FACIAL PARALYSIS)

In this condition, the facial nerve on one side of the face suddenly becomes inflamed and swollen. It is possible that this may be a reaction to a viral infection, but the exact cause is unknown. Eighty five per cent of patients recover completely but recovery can be a long process and it may take nine months or more before the nerve is working normally again.

Let us suppose that a forty five year old woman has come to the acupuncture clinic with a left-sided Bell's palsy. She has all the usual signs of this condition: an inability to shut the eye completely on the affected side, watering of that eye, drooping of the left corner of her mouth, and a paralysis of the facial muscles on the left side so that she can no longer smile, frown or purse her lips. On examination, the left side of her face appears slightly swollen, as does the area around her left eye. Her tongue has a white coating, and her pulse is superficial in character and slow. As with all patients suffering from this condition, she says that it came on rapidly, over the course of a day or two.

In Chinese medicine, paralysis of any type is attributed to a complete blockage of the flow of *qi* and of blood. The suddenness of this attack's onset suggests that it was due to an invasion by wind. This diagnosis is supported by the puffiness of the patient's face and eye. The white coating on her tongue and her slow pulse indicate that cold has also been a factor in producing the obstruction of qi. The aim of treatment, therefore, is to disperse the wind and cold, and to stimulate the circulation of blood and of qi. Moxa may be used to warm the points.

Table 16 shows a selection of the many points that may be used in the treatment of this condition.

TABLE 16: TREATMENT OF A PATIENT WITH BELL'S PALSY

Point	Name	Meaning	Location	Action
St 2	Sibai	Brightness in four directions	On the cheekbone, on a line running vertically down through the midpoint of the eye	Eliminates wind; is said to improve the eyesight in all four directions
St 4	Dicang	Storehouse of Earth	At the corner of the mouth	A local point specific for the treatment of facial paralysis
SJ 17	Yifeng	Wind shield	In the depression behind the base of the ear	An important point for treating problems of the face and head; eliminates wind
GB 1	Tong-ziliao	Pupil opening	In the depression next to the outer angle of the eye	Eliminates wind
GB 2	Tinghui	Gathering of hearing	Just in front of the ear, at the joint of the jaw	A local point specific for the treatment of facial paralysis
GB 12	Wangu	Mastoid bone	In the depression behind the ear, behind and below the mastoid bone	A local point specific for the treatment of facial paralysis
GB 20	Fengchi	Windpool	At the back of the neck, in the depression below the base of the skull	May be an *ah-shi* point in this condition; an important point for eliminating wind and cold

HEATSTROKE

This is one condition where Western medicine and Chinese medicine agree about the cause. The Western doctor will say it is caused by heat, especially when the atmosphere is humid, preventing the patient from cooling down through the evaporation of sweat. The Chinese physician will say much the same thing – it is caused by an invasion of summer heat, which is a fierce, damp heat.

If we picture a patient with this condition, he is flushed, thirsty and slightly confused, and he has a headache. His mouth is dry and his pulse is superficial, bounding in character and rapid. The signs all point to invasion by heat, and the patient's confusion suggests that his heart (the seat of the mind) has been affected. The treatment is to disperse the heat.

Some of the points that might be used are shown in table 17.

TABLE 17: TREATMENT OF A PATIENT WITH HEATSTROKE

Point	Name	Meaning	Location	Action
LI 4	Hegu	Valley junction	On the back of the hand, in the angle between the thumb and forefinger	Eliminates heat; tranquilises the mind
St 36	Zusanli	Three *li* (or *cun*) on the legs	Three *li* (or *cun*) below the knee	Strengthens *qi*, nourishes *yin*, counteracts the effect of summer heat
UB 40	Weizhong	Crooked centre	At the centre of the crease behind the knee	If the point is pricked to make it bleed, helps to eliminate heat, stimulate the flow of blood, and restore consciousness
P 6	Neiguan	Medial pass	A little way above the crease on the front of the wrist, on the midline of the forearm	Can be pricked to eliminate heat
P 7	Daling	Large mound	In the middle of the crease on the front of the wrist	Has a similar function to P 5 and can be used with it to reinforce its effect
P 8	Laogong	Centre of work	In the centre of the palm of the hand	Has a similar function to P 6 and can be used with it to reinforce its effect

GASTROENTERITIS

This is another condition that can often affect people who are visiting hot countries. Let us say that the patient is a young man who is having a two week holiday in Spain. After a couple of days, he has developed abdominal pain and is passing hot, yellow, loose and smelly stools that burn his anus as he passes them. He has a slight fever and is sweating. He has vomited a couple of times and, although he does not feel able to eat, he keeps on drinking water because he is thirsty most of the time. He has a sweet taste in his mouth that the water does not wash away. On examination, his face is flushed and his lips are dry, despite his intake of water. His tongue is red with a sticky yellow coating, and his pulse is rapid with a slippery or gliding quality to it.

The passage of smelly, loose, yellow stools is indicative of an invasion of the spleen, stomach and intestines by damp heat. As a result, the normal extraction of *qi* from food by the stomach and spleen has been disrupted and the circulation of *qi* has become disordered. The fever and thirst, together with the patient's flushed face and red tongue, confirm the involvement of heat. A sweet taste in the mouth is associated with problems in the Earth organs – the stomach and spleen – and their meridians, while dry lips are also indicative of heat in the spleen. A rapid pulse, of course, signifies heat, while its forceful, slippery quality implies an invasion of the digestive tract by damp, which is blocking the digestive process. Treatment aims to eliminate the damp heat and restore the stomach, spleen and intestines to normal working order.

Table 18 shows some of the points that might be used to treat this patient.

TABLE 18: TREATMENT OF A PATIENT WITH GASTROENTERITIS

Point	Name	Meaning	Location	Action
LI 4	Hegu	Valley junction	On the back of the hand, in the angle between the thumb and forefinger	Eliminates heat
St 25	Tianshu	Pivot of heaven	On the abdomen, lying between the region above the umbilicus (pertaining to heaven and *yang*) and that below it (pertaining to earth and *yin*)	Regulates the function of the stomach and intestines by eliminating damp and strengthening *qi*
Sp 9	Yinling-quan	Yin hill spring	On the medial aspect of the leg, just below the knee	Eliminates damp; strengthens the spleen
UB 25	Dach-angshu	Large intestine *shu* point	Lateral to the spine, at about the level of the top of the hip bone	Stimulates the large intestine and its meridian
P 6	Neiguan	Medial pass	A little way above the crease on the front of the wrist, on the midline of the forearm	Eliminates heat; acts through its association with its fellow Fire meridian, the Sanjiao, whose middle section contains the stomach and spleen
Ren 12	Zhong-wan	Middle of stomach	On the midline of the abdomen, a little way above the umbilicus	The *mu*, or alarm, point of the stomach, used to eliminate heat and damp from the stomach and spleen

BED WETTING

All children who wet the bed grow out of the habit eventually, but some take longer than others. When the condition continues beyond the age of three or four, it can become a serious problem, not only to the parents who have to change and wash the sheets, but also to the child who may become very anxious about his inability to stop. There are various Western treatments available. A popular one is to use an electronic buzzer that is sensitive to damp. As soon as the child starts to wet the bed, the buzzer goes off and wakes him up. Some children find this very effective and, eventually, start to wake naturally, as soon as they feel they need to urinate. For children who don't respond, medication may be prescribed. The first of these is desmopressin, which reduces the amount of urine produced by the kidneys during the night and is usually prescribed for periods of three to six months. Alternatively, there is a group of preparations known as anticholinergic drugs which reduce the sensitivity of the bladder, thus helping it to stretch more and hold more urine. Drugs only tend to be recommended if other forms of treatment have failed.

However, for those children whose parents don't want them to take drugs, and for those who don't respond to orthodox treatments, acupuncture may prove very useful.

In Chinese medicine, bed wetting is seen as a lack of control over the urine due to a deficiency in the Water (Kidney and Urinary Bladder) meridians, and treatment is aimed at strengthening these. Interestingly, the drug desmopressin also works by counteracting a deficiency – in this case, of the naturally occurring antidiuretic hormone (ADH) which, in most people, is produced by the brain during sleep and reduces the amount of urine produced by the kidneys. Children who wet the bed may not experience this natural surge of hormone and so desmopressin can remedy the deficiency.

Table 19 shows some of the points that could be used to treat a child with bed wetting.

TABLE 19: TREATMENT OF A CHILD WHO WETS THE BED

Point	Name	Meaning	Location	Action
UB 23	Shenshu	Kidney *shu* point	To the side of the spine, at about the level of the waist	Stimulates the functional *qi* of the kidney; a major point for treating disorders of the urinary tract
UB 28	Pang-guang-shu	Bladder *shu* point	To the side of the spine, in the sacral region (the hip area)	Strengthens the *qi* of the bladder
Ren 3	Zhongji	Exact centre	At the 'centre' of the body, on the midline of the abdomen, a short way above the pubic bone	A major point for treating disorders of the urinary tract
Ren 4	Guan-yuan	Storage place of *qi*	On the midline of the abdomen, above Ren 3	Strengthens the kidney
Ren 6	Qihai	Sea of *qi*	On the abdomen, on the midline, above Ren 4 and a little way below the umbilicus	Strengthens the kidney

IMPOTENCE

This is another condition in which the kidney is involved. In Chinese medicine, the kidney is believed to be responsible for governing the reproductive system, so any abnormalities in a patient's sexual function are said to stem from problems relating to the kidney. Since impotence may be seen as a form of deficiency, with aspects of internalisation and lack of movement, the element that would be deficient is yang, resulting in a relative excess of yin. The deficiency may involve not only the Kidney meridian but also the Ren meridian (or Vessel of Conception), the midline channel running down the front of the body. The Ren meridian is associated with the sexual organs because of its pathway. Treatment of impotence consists primarily of stimulating the *yang* of the kidney in order to restore balance.

Possible points for the treatment of impotence are shown in table 20.

TABLE 20: TREATMENT OF A MAN WITH IMPOTENCE

Point	Name	Meaning	Location	Action
UB 23	Shenshu	Kidney *shu* point	To the side of the spine, at about the level of the waist	Stimulates the functional *qi* of the kidney; a major point for treating disorders of the urogenital system
Du 4	Mingmen	Door of life	On the midline of the back, at the level of the kidney, whose *qi* is the basic source for the whole body	Stimulates the functional *qi* of the kidney; an important point for reinforcing the *yang* of the kidney
Du 20	Baihui	A hundred meetings	At the crossing point of the Urinary Bladder, Liver and Du meridians, on the crown of the head	Regulates and activates *yang qi*
Ren 3	Zhongji	Exact centre	At the 'centre' of the body, on the midline of the abdomen, a short way above the pubic bone	A major point for treating disorders of the urogenital system; used for its direct effect on the kidney
Ren 4	Guan-yuan	Storage place of *qi*	On the midline of the abdomen, above Ren 3	Strengthens the kidney; moxi-bustion of this point strengthens the *yang* of the kidney

FEBRILE CONVULSIONS

Some children are prone to have fits if they develop infections that cause their temperatures to rise rapidly. Fortunately, it is a susceptibility that most grow out of after the age of about two, and usually the fits are short-lived and therefore not life-threatening. But, naturally, they are extremely worrying for the parents.

Let us imagine an eighteen month old girl who, having caught a cold a few days previously, has suddenly developed a high fever and had a fit, during which she has gone blue for a few seconds. On examination following the fit, she is flushed and has a rapid pulse that feels wiry. A sudden onset of disease always suggests the involvement of wind, while the fever and rapid pulse indicate the presence of heat. Cyanosis (going blue) suggests that the liver is involved, since this is the organ responsible for the normal circulation of qi. The treatment is to eliminate both heat and wind, which can be effected by using some of the points shown in table 21. Naturally, when treating a small child, the number of needles is kept to a minimum. The points described here would never be used all at the same time.

TABLE 21: TREATMENT OF A CHILD WITH FEBRILE CONVULSIONS

Point	Name	Meaning	Location	Action
LI 1	Shang-yang	*Yang shang* (*shang* is the sound associated with Metal and its meridians)	On the thumb side of the index finger, near the corner of the nail	Eliminates wind
LI 4	Hegu	Valley junction	On the back of the hand, in the angle between the thumb and forefinger	Eliminates heat; clears obstructions to the flow of *qi*; specific point for relieving convulsions; tranquilises the mind
LI 11	Quchi	Crooked pool	In a depression at the lateral side of the elbow crease	Eliminates heat and wind; an important point for the treatment of fever
SI 3	Houxi	Back brook	In a depression on the little finger side of the hand, just above the line of the knuckles	Eliminates heat; relieves spasm by tranquilising the mind
K 1	Yong-quan	Gushing spring	In the depression on the sole of the foot, from where the *qi* of the meridian gushes upwards	An important point for treating infantile convulsions of any kind
P 8	Laogong	Centre of work	In the centre of the palm of the hand	Eliminates heat; relieves spasm by tranquilising the mind
GB 34	Yangling-quan	*Yang* mound spring	In a depression below the bony prominence on the lateral aspect of the knee	Promotes the flow of *qi*; eliminates wind and heat; an important point for treating infantile convulsions
Liv 2	Xingjian	Walking in the middle	Between the first and second toes	Eliminates heat from the liver to prevent wind from being generated internally
Liv 3	Taichong	Great pass	On the upper aspect of the foot, on a line that runs between the first and second toes	Eliminates heat from the liver to prevent wind from being generated internally

NOSEBLEEDS

Some people are troubled by recurrent nosebleeds. Usually the bleeding occurs from an area at the back of the nose, known as Little's area, which is particularly well supplied with tiny blood vessels. These vessels may become fragile and bleed at the slightest provocation. If the nosebleeds become very frequent or severe, Western medicine offers cauterisation of Little's area. This is a fairly minor procedure which usually stops further bleeding.

However, let us look at a patient who has not tried Western treatment and who has arrived at the acupuncture clinic just after having had a nosebleed. On examination, he looks slightly flushed, and his pulse is rapid. Haemorrhage is often due to invasion by heat. The nose is the sense organ that is associated with the lungs, so we can deduce from the patient's symptoms that there is an excess of heat in the Lung meridian. This is corroborated by the patient's pulse and his flushed appearance. Treatment consists of eradicating the heat.

Table 22 shows some of the points that might be used.

TABLE 22: TREATMENT OF A PATIENT WITH NOSEBLEEDS

Point	Name	Meaning	Location	Action
Lu 11	Shao-shang	Lesser *shang* (*shang* is the sound associated with Metal and its meridians)	Near the corner of the thumbnail	Eliminates heat from the lung
LI 4	Hegu	Valley junction	On the back of the hand, in the angle between the thumb and forefinger	An important point for treating diseases of the lung (the Large Intestine and Lung meridians are both Metal, so they have a close affinity); eliminates heat from the lung
UB 60	Kunlun	A mountain in Tibet	On the lateral aspect of the ankle, between the Achilles tendon and the ankle bone	Eliminates heat from the lung*
K 3	Taixi	Great canyon	On the medial aspect of the ankle, in the depression beside the Achilles tendon	Eliminates heat from the lung*

**The combination of UB 60 and K 3 can be used to stop a nosebleed which has been brought on by heat arising as a result of a relative excess of yang caused by a deficiency of kidney yin. These points can be used as a first aid measure to stop a nosebleed, since pressure on the two points works just as well as needling. An acupuncturist may instruct his patient on the exact location of these points for emergency use.*

SOME CASE HISTORIES

Several of the following case histories are included here with the kind permission of Mr. Roger Murray of Lewes, Sussex, the late Dr. Peter Helps of Brighton, Sussex, and, of course, their patients.

GABRIELLE

This middle-aged woman first saw an acupuncturist during the month of February. The previous September, she had stretched her right arm back to pick something up and had felt a tearing pain in her shoulder. It had subsided after a few minutes and she thought no more of it until it started up again some days later, this time lasting for three weeks. After this, she was free of pain until November, when it returned and gradually became worse, spreading to affect her upper arm as well. She was unable to lie on her right side at night. If she stretched her arm above her head while she was asleep, the pain would wake her up, sweating and gasping for breath.

Gabrielle went to see her doctor and was told that she had a frozen shoulder. The doctor added that there was little that he could offer in the way of treatment. Steroid injections or manipulation under anaesthetic were sometimes used but, in some cases, these had been known to make matters worse. If left alone, the condition should resolve itself in about two years, so his advice was to take painkillers and wait.

Gabrielle worked as a librarian in the local university library, so she had to be able to lift heavy books and sometimes put them onto high shelves. Since she could no longer raise her arm higher than the horizontal, she could not do her job. She could not have two years' sick leave – either she had to find a cure or lose her job. One of her friends recommended an acupuncturist, to whom she went with some trepidation.

On examination, Gabrielle was found to have a wiry pulse, indicating a stagnation of blood and of qi. Because of the location of the pain, a diagnosis was made of stagnation in the Large Intestine, Small Intestine and Sanjiao meridians. Gabrielle's tongue had cracks in the centre and at the sides, suggesting a *yin* deficiency. In all, Gabrielle had eight sessions of treatment, during which the points detailed in table 23 were used.

At the first session, the acupuncturist used three local points to treat the pain

– SJ 14, LI 15 and SI 10, two points to move the stagnation – LI 4 and SJ 5, and one – Sp 6 – to treat the *yin* deficiency. Gabrielle was asked to return at weekly intervals.

At her next appointment, Gabrielle reported that the pain was not quite so bad, and she was sleeping a little better. On examination, her pulse was found to be less wiry. The acupuncturist used the same points as before, together with an additional local point, LI 16. The problem seemed to be due to an external rather than an internal disharmony, and it was to resolve this that the main treatment was aimed.

The following week, Gabrielle reported that, although the pain was less severe, she had had a menstrual period that lasted for twelve days. Her pulse was found to be deficient. Because *qi* is extracted and refined from the air in the lungs, Lung meridian points can be used to nourish the whole body. In states of Lung meridian deficiency, the shoulder is especially vulnerable to problems. Because there was now a suggestion of an internal Lung deficiency, some points were used to nourish the interior, although the main treatment was still external. The local points treated were Lu 2, SI 10 and SJ 14. Needles were also put in the distal points Lu 7 and K 6.

By the next appointment, Gabrielle was feeling much better and was finding it easier to move her arm. She had also noticed that the athlete's foot that she had had for many years was beginning to clear up. The treatment from the previous week was repeated, with the addition of LI 16.

On her fifth visit, Gabrielle was found to have a 'soggy' pulse and a thin white coating on her tongue, both indicating the presence of damp heat. The previous treatment was repeated, together with a needle in GB 34.

By April, Gabrielle was reporting more good days than bad. The pain that had originally been sharp (indicating a stagnation of blood) had given way to a dull ache (indicating a stagnation of qi). This was a definite improvement because stagnation of blood is seen as being a symptom of a deeper disharmony than stagnation of qi. The pain was no longer in one place but tended to move around, suggesting invasion by wind, which classically affects the two Wood meridians,

Liver and Gall Bladder. To remedy this, a local point, GB 21, and a distal point, GB 34, were used in addition to the regular treatment.

By May, after eight sessions with the acupuncturist, Gabrielle was free from pain, had regained almost all the movement in her arm, and was able to return to work.

TABLE 23: GABRIELLE'S TREATMENT

Point	Name	Meaning	Location	Action
Lu 2	Yunmen	Cloud door	In the hollow below the outer end of the collarbone	Used for its local effect on the shoulder
Lu 7	Lieque	Broken clouds	On the thumb side of the wrist, above the bony prominence	Activates and strengthens the *qi* of the lung
LI 4	Hegu	Valley junction	On the back of the hand, in the angle between the thumb and forefinger	Clears obstructions to the flow of *qi*; relieves pain and weakness in the hands and arms
LI 15	Jianyu	Corner of shoulder	Just below the point of the shoulder	Specific for pain in the shoulder joint
LI 16	Jugu	Huge bone (the ancient Chinese name for the collarbone)	On the ridge of the shoulder	Used for its local effect on the shoulder
Sp 6	Sanyin-jiao	Three *yin* meridians crossing	At the intersection point of the Spleen, Liver and Kidney meridians, on the medial aspect of the leg, a short way above the ankle	Stimulates and nourishes *yin*
SI 10	Naoshu	Point at muscle prominence	At the back of the shoulder joint	Specific for pain in the shoulder joint
K 6	Zhaohai	Shining sea	On the inner aspect of the ankle	Opens the *yin* Ren meridian to help counteract *yin* deficiency
SJ 5	Waiguan	Lateral pass	Just above the wrist, on the lateral side of the humerus	Relieves stagnation of *qi*
SJ 14	Jianliao	Shoulder opening	In a hollow below the bone at the back of the shoulder	Specific for pain in the shoulder joint
GB 21	Jianjing	Well of the shoulder	Where the base of the neck joins the shoulder	Specific for pain in the shoulder joint
GB 34	Yangling-quan	*Yang* mound spring	In a depression below the bony prominence on the lateral aspect of the knee	Stimulates *qi*; relieves obstruction; eliminates wind and damp heat; stimulates liver *yin**

**Liver yin nourishes the joints so, by improving this, mobility is improved.*

CATHERINE

Catherine was a menopausal woman who went to see an acupuncturist for the first time during a heat wave in August. She had been having hot flushes for some time and, up till then, they had not troubled her too much but, since the heat wave had begun, she had been finding them intolerable.

At the menopause, there is said to be a decline in the body's jing, or essence. Jing is one of the so-called 'three treasures' of Chinese medicine, the others being shen (spirit) and qi. Jing is said to regulate the whole cycle of growth, maturation and decline. When it begins to decrease around the menopause, it sets up an imbalance between *yin* and yang. Hot flushes (particularly at night, when *yin* should be at its strongest) are a manifestation of excessive yang, as is the restlessness that they usually cause.

On examination, Catherine's tongue showed cracks, suggesting a *yin* deficiency, and her pulse was deficient at the deep levels, indicating a deficiency in the interior, yin, organs. Catherine had four sessions of treatment during which the points detailed in table 24 were used.

After two sessions, Catherine was much better. Two further sessions at six-monthly intervals were all she needed to see her through the menopause.

TABLE 24: CATHERINE'S TREATMENT

Point	Name	Meaning	Location	Action
Lu 7	Lieque	Broken clouds	On the thumb side of the wrist, above the bony prominence	Strengthens *qi*, nourishes *yin*
St 36	Zusanli	Three *li* (or *cun*) on the legs	Three *li* (or *cun*) below the knee	Strengthens *qi*, nourishes *yin*
Sp 6	Sanyin-jiao	Three *yin* meridians crossing	At the intersection point of the Spleen, Liver and Kidney meridians, on the medial aspect of the leg, a short way above the ankle	Nourishes *yin*
K 6	Zhaohai	Shining sea	On the inner aspect of the ankle	Opens the *yin* Ren meridian to help counteract *yin* deficiency by making the *yin* in the Ren meridian available to the rest of the body

BRIAN

This twenty four year old man woke one morning to find that he was unable to move his right wrist. He could use his arm perfectly normally but his right hand hung limply and could not be raised. This condition, known as wrist drop, is usually due to injury or prolonged pressure affecting the nerve supply to the muscles of the forearm and hand. However, in Brian's case, no such history was forthcoming.

He was referred by his GP to the neurology specialist at the local hospital and a diagnosis of localised nerve damage was made. The only explanation seemed to be that Brian had lain in such a position while asleep that the nerve was stretched or damaged.

Whatever, the cause, though, the neurologist told him that there was no specific treatment – he would just have to wait for the nerve to recover, something that could take between six months and two years. Meanwhile, he was to have physiotherapy to prevent the affected muscles from contracting.

It was the physiotherapist who suggested that acupuncture might help, and Brian decided to go for treatment.

TABLE 25: BRIAN'S TREATMENT

Point	Name	Meaning	Location	Action
Lu 7	Lieque	Broken clouds	On the thumb side of the wrist, above the bony prominence	Eliminates wind; a specific point for treating weakness or paralysis in the wrist
LI 4	Hegu	Valley junction	On the back of the hand, in the angle between the thumb and forefinger	Eliminates wind; clears obstruction to the flow of *qi*
SI 4	Wangu	Wrist bone	On the side of the wrist, above the little finger	A specific point for treating weakness or paralysis of the wrist
SJ 4	Yangchi	Pool of *yang*	On the back of the wrist	Stimulates the flow of *qi* and removes obstructions; also used for its local effects on the hand and wrist
SJ 5	Waiguan	Lateral pass	Just above the wrist, a short distance above SJ 4, on the lateral side of the humerus	Relieves stagnation of *qi*

A sudden paralysis of this nature suggests an obstruction to the flow of *qi* due to invasion by wind. The acupuncturist used local points around the wrist to eliminate the wind and cl, as shown in table 25.

Brian was treated every other day for two weeks, after which time he had recovered a considerable amount of movement in his wrist. He continued to have treatment twice a week and, within six weeks was back to normal.

JAMES

James was a forty three year old man who, twenty years earlier, having taken a degree in geology at London University, was offered a job with a large firm in Australia. He leaped at the chance of seeing the world and undertook his new job with great enthusiasm.

For a time, everything went very well. He was competent and well-liked by the people with whom he worked, and he met and subsequently got engaged to an Australian woman. However, one day there was a very bad accident at his worksite which resulted in two men being seriously injured.

It fell to James to write out the reports of these accidents and, while he was doing so, his right arm suddenly stopped functioning. He could grip the pen with his hand but was quite unable to move his arm. He saw the company doctor who was unable to explain what had happened.

After several weeks there was no sign of recovery and, eventually, James lost his job on the grounds of chronic incapacity. He was thoroughly depressed by this and, even more so, by the fact that no one could tell him what had caused the problem or whether it was ever likely to get better. He was unable to face searching for another job in a country that was not his home so, breaking off his engagement, he left for England.

Back home, his incapacity made it hard to get a job and he had to take whatever he could get. He remained unsettled. His arm was not improving, and the muscles were beginning to shrivel. After a succession of jobs that offered him no mental challenge, he decided to start his own business. It was around this time, too, that he met an English woman and married her.

But he continued to be dogged by bad luck. Eventually, his business capsized and he was left with serious financial problems. He struggled on but was having difficulties at home as well. Finally, he and his wife divorced. He found a job but, as before, it was no challenge to him. This, together with his divorce and financial problems, produced a severe depression, and he became suicidal.

It was at this point that a friend suggested to him that he have some acupuncture treatment. The acupuncturist he went to was a practitioner of the Five Elements school. Based on the fact that James' face appeared to have yellow lines, his voice was singing in character, and he craved sympathy, the acupuncturist diagnosed an imbalance in his Earth meridians. In addition, the acupuncturist noted James' great interest in geology and things of the earth. The Earth meridians are those of the Spleen and the Stomach. On taking James's pulses, the two corresponding to these meridians were found to be bounding.

The treatment comprised sedation of the meridians that were in excess, together with transfer of *qi* from them to deficient meridians by the use of specific transfer points. In addition, the source points (see chapter 6) of the Stomach and Spleen meridians were used, because these are the direct links to the stomach and spleen themselves. The element points – that is, the Earth points – on both meridians were also used (see chapter 3).

After two months of treatment, although there was as yet no noticeable difference in his arm, James' whole attitude towards life started to change. The depression left him and he started to think in a far more positive manner than before. He began to talk about returning to Australia to see if he could find his fiancée of twenty years before.

After four months, he started to regain some movement in his arm and was referred by his general practitioner to the local hospital for physiotherapy.

After nine months of treatment, James returned to Australia. Two months later, his acupuncturist received a letter saying that he had met up again with his first fiancée. She had married a year after he had left Australia but her marriage, too, had failed. They were intending to get married shortly. James' arm was continuing to improve and he was hoping to find an acupuncturist in Adelaide, where they were settling, in order to continue treatment.

DEREK

This forty five year old man telephoned the acupuncture clinic one Thursday afternoon, asking for an emergency appointment. He had severe toothache and needed some treatment to control the pain until he could see his dentist on the following Monday morning.

His history was an interesting one. He had been a high-powered executive in a large company for a number of years, and the pressures under which he worked were enormous. His sphere of responsibility gradually increased until, to relieve the stress, he started to drink. His alcohol intake increased until he was drinking a bottle of whisky, or more, a day. By this time, it was the alcohol that was making it impossible for him to cope with his job, and he was replaced.

After this trauma, he found another job and managed to stop drinking with the aid of Alcoholics Anonymous, but his body began to react to all the various stresses that he had been under and he started to develop allergies. At first, he reacted only to common allergens such as pollen and cat fur. But then, he began to find that certain foods would make him vomit. Finally, chemical compounds such as diesel fumes began to affect him, so that he was unable to walk along a busy road without feeling sick and faint.

He went to see a specialist at the local hospital and was started on a course of desensitising injections. He was warned that the course of treatment could be a long one, since he seemed to be allergic to so many substances.

Not long after this, Derek developed toothache. Now, this case occurred some decades ago when general anaesthesia was still being used regularly by dentists and, although the toothache was quite severe, Derek knew that he would be unable to visit the dentist immediately because he would be affected by the anaesthetic gases that had built up in the air of the dental surgery during the week. The only answer was to get an appointment for first thing on Monday morning, when the surgery would be relatively gas-free. Meanwhile, he needed something to control the pain – and that was when he contacted the acupuncturist.

However, although acupuncture can be used for emergency treatment, the best results are achieved when a course of treatment is given. And while it is perfectly possible to obtain relief from symptoms after a single session, the fact that acupuncture works by manipulating energies means that problems may occur at a later date if the energies are not completely returned to normal. So when Derek called to request an emergency appointment, he was told that he could only be seen if he agreed to come for a follow-up course of treatment.

Derek agreed to this, and his toothache was treated by the insertion of two needles. The pain was relieved and, on the following Monday, he saw his dentist. When he returned to the acupuncturist to start his course of treatment, a diagnosis was made according to the Law of the Five Elements. Derek showed grief and anguish when he spoke about his problems and his voice had a weeping quality, indicating that the element that was out of balance was Metal. However, his face had a bluish look to it and his bodily smell seemed putrid, suggesting that there were problems with the Water element as well. The acupuncturist diagnosed a deficiency in both elements. As we saw in chapter 3, a deficiency in the mother element will lead to an undernourished child element – the so-called screaming child syndrome. In this case, a deficiency in Metal had resulted in a deficiency in Water, which is its child.

The treatment consisted of stimulating the deficient Metal using primarily the element points (that is, the Metal points on the two Metal meridians, the Large Intestine and the Lung) and also the source points on the Metal meridians.

By his fourth treatment, there had been a noticeable improvement and the consultant at the hospital suggested that Derek's allergy injections should be gradually reduced. After four months of acupuncture treatment, the injections were stopped altogether as all traces of the allergies had disappeared.

PAUL

Paul was a thirty two year old policeman who had joined the force some eight years earlier, after coming out of the Army. Although he enjoyed his job, he found it stressful.

Paul had coped with a number of fairly traumatic incidents in his earlier life, including involvement in a very severe accident at the age of twenty one when he was knocked off his motorcycle. He had been in intensive care for three months following this but ultimately made a full recovery and was able to return to his Army duties. However, when he was twenty five, during an overseas posting, he had seen a friend badly injured and had, himself, narrowly escaped being killed.

All this stress had taken its toll, and Paul had become a chain smoker. And, although his job with the police force was far less stressful than his previous work, he had much less resistance than before. He started to have recurrent attacks of severe pain in his chest and back, accompanied by shivering. On two occasions he had been rushed to hospital with a suspected heart attack. He described himself as being full of fear.

It was becoming clear to Paul that, sooner or later, he would not be able to carry on with his job. He decided to seek some help and, on the advice of a colleague, made an appointment for some acupuncture, with the idea of trying to get rid of his chest pain.

He was diagnosed, in accordance with the Law of the Five Elements, as having problems relating to Metal. This was based on the weeping quality of his voice, the anguish and grief with which he told his story, the white appearance of his face, and his rotten body smell. However, he also appeared to be suffering from a complete obstruction to the circulation of *qi*. So the acupuncturist decided to use a very powerful combination of needles known as the Treatment of the Seven Dragons which is used specifically in cases of severe disruption of the energy flow affecting the whole body. After the treatment, Paul started to tremble. This became quite severe and lasted for about forty five minutes after the needles had been removed.

Follow-up treatments consisted of strengthening the heart and the Heart meridian. The heart is associated with Fire, and Metal is the servant of fire, so weakness of Fire can result in it losing control of Metal. Because of this, the Metal source points and element points were also used.

The results were remarkable. After only a few treatments, Paul was starting to feel better and was much less fearful. After several months he had lost all his anxiety and was enjoying life to the full.

8

ACUPUNCTURE AND MODERN SCIENCE

When this book was first published in 1987, the first paragraph of this chapter began:

> *We live today in a scientific and materialistic world in which miracles don't happen – or, if they do, they must be explained or disproved. In the last few decades, science has developed to such an extent that everything now has to be proved scientifically in order to be acceptable. All too often science has made it impossible for us to accept something which cannot be readily explained in its own terms, and charlatans and forgers over the years have helped to make sceptics of us all. Complementary medicine has suffered greatly in this respect. To those of us who have been brought up in the West, in an environment of hospitals and health services, the complementary therapies, particularly some of the rather more 'way out' ones, seem to be in much the same category as fortune telling and UFOs.*

But, in the years since then, things have changed dramatically. As patients have discovered how helpful complementary therapies can be either instead of orthodox medicine or as an adjunct to it, they have voted with their feet – and have recommended their practitioners to others. Doctors, too, have changed in their attitude – nowadays, it seems that they are far more likely to be sympathetic to complementary therapies than to condemn them. And, although it's not easy to get accurate figures to reflect the numbers of people using complementary therapies, the information that is available shows a steady increase. In 2008 the Nursing Times reported that *"Complementary and alternative medicine (CAM) has grown rapidly [in the UK] over the last two decades and is now used by around six million people a year"*. By 2017 the College of Medicine and Integrated Health was putting that figure at around 9 million – an increase of 50 per cent in nine years. Nowadays most British towns – and many villages – have one or more complementary practitioners working there.

'Scientific' proof has become less necessary. Anyone who has taken the time to investigate acupuncture will tell you that there is no doubt that it works. And patients who have been treated with acupuncture and consequently recovered from conditions for which Western practitioners have little to offer will tell you that they don't care how it works. Acupuncture has been proving its worth for two thousand years – scientific investigation of its workings should not be deemed essential in order to corroborate this fact.

Over the years, investigations into acupuncture have been carried out in the West, many of them based on the premise that it is the anatomically demonstrable nervous system, rather than the hypothetical system of meridians, that is responsible for the results achieved by the therapy. It must be said, however, that physicians still do not fully understand the workings of the nervous system. So scientific experiments designed to demonstrate pseudo-acupuncture effects are doing so only in the light of an incompletely understood system.

However, it can do no harm to ask how acupuncture is related to physiology as understood by Western physicians, although many of the experiments to investigate acupuncture have been performed on animals (a highly controversial issue in itself). These have shown that stimulation of certain points on the skin can produce effects at a distance from these points, and these effects seem to be dependent on the normal functioning of the nervous system. Because animal experimentation permits the destruction of various parts of the animal's nervous system, it has also been possible to find out which part of the system carries the signal. What is interesting is that experiments trying to investigate the nervous system theory of acupuncture seem to show that the nervous impulses supposedly responsible for producing the effects appear to be carried in different ways. It is therefore difficult to propound an overall theory explaining in Western terms how acupuncture works.

Experiments have been performed in which stimulation of the skin on the back of rats produced changes in their intestines. The results were found to be the same whether a rat's nervous system was intact or its spinal cord had been divided, cutting off the body from the brain. From this it was deduced that the brain was not involved in the process and that all the nervous impulses controlling the effects of stimulation were carried by the spinal cord. However, a similar experiment performed on fish, where stimulation of the skin produced changes in the lower part of the bowel, was found to be effective even if the spinal cord had been destroyed. In this case, a different mechanism seemed to be involved, the effects apparently being produced by the sympathetic nervous system.

In his book *Acupuncture: The Ancient Chinese Art of Healing* (Heinemann 1962), Felix Mann put forward the theory that the responses obtained in various organs of the body when points on the skin are stimulated tie in with the way in which the body develops as an embryo. Each section of the body, together with its nerve supply, develops from a different section of the embryo. Physicians call these sections dermatomes. Very often, both an organ and the acupuncture points that affect it lie in the same dermatome. However, Mann pointed out that *"the acupuncture points of the legs and head do not fit in with what is known of dermatomes"*. So another theory would need to be found to explain how acupuncture works in these parts of the body – and, indeed, why they should be different from the rest.

The discovery of endorphins in the 1970s helped many previously sceptical doctors to accept acupuncture as a method of pain relief. Endorphins are substances produced by the body that have the effect of controlling pain. Secretion of large amounts of endorphins occurs automatically in response to trauma which is why, for example, a seriously injured person may feel little or no pain immediately after the injury. It would appear that the level of endorphins circulating in the bloodstream under normal conditions varies from person to person. This may explain why different people have different pain thresholds, some being able to tolerate pain far more readily than others.

Stimulation of acupuncture points that produce anaesthetic effects has been shown to release endorphins into the body. What has not been explained – at least, not in Western terms – is why stimulation of these particular points and no others produces these effects.

There are, of course, many studies, set up to assess the value of acupuncture in the treatment of individual conditions, that have proved to the experimenter's satisfaction that the therapy doesn't work. However, reading these studies, it is quite clear that the experimenters do not understand how acupuncture has to be used. It is no good taking a random selection of patients suffering from asthma and using the same three acupuncture points to treat them all. As we saw in the previous chapter, asthma can be caused by a number of quite different factors according to Chinese theory, and they need to be treated in different ways. Acupuncture is a holistic therapy, treating the patient, not the disease. And scientific methods and randomized controlled trials cannot be used with therapies such as this, where the treatment is chosen specifically for that individual patient.

9

ON TREATMENT AND TRAINING

FINDING AN ACUPUNCTURIST

If you're looking for an acupuncturist, it's important to find someone who is fully qualified and registered. Some practitioners of other complementary therapies and, indeed, some doctors will offer acupuncture to their patients, but few of them will have done the full three or four years of training that a registered acupuncturist will have undertaken. This means that, while these other therapists and doctors may be perfectly competent when it comes to using acupuncture needles to treat localised pain or inserting ear studs to help with giving up smoking or dieting, that is the limit of their expertise.

However, thanks to the internet, it is now much easier than it used to be to find a fully qualified and registered practitioner.

In the UK, the holder of the register is the British Acupuncture Council (BAcC):

https://acupuncture.org.uk/find-an-acupuncturist/

You can also 'phone the Council on 020 8735 0400.

In the USA, the National Certification Commission for Acupuncture and Oriental Medicine (NCCAOM) has 20,390 board certified acupuncturists on its register:

https://directory.nccaom.org/

In Australia, acupuncturists are regulated by the Chinese Medicine Board of Australia (CMBA) and a register of practitioners is held by the Australian Acupuncture & Chinese Medicine Association (AACMA):

https://www.acupuncture.org.au/find-a-practitioner

HAVING TREATMENT

It is important to remember that, like any therapy, acupuncture doesn't work every time (although this doesn't mean that if it didn't work for you with one set of symptoms in the past it won't work for you with a different set of symptoms now). In addition, depending on how long you have had your symptoms, it may take a while before you begin to notice any great improvement, so it is important to be patient and not give up on your treatments. But if the therapy is going to work, you are likely to see some improvement in your condition by the fourth or fifth treatment (you may, of course, start to feel better after the first session). Once you do start to improve, it is very important to keep up with the treatment until the acupuncturist says you can stop. This goes back to the business of balancing energies. The first few treatments will start qi flowing normally again but, if treatment is not continued, there is a danger that you could relapse, leaving your qi just as unbalanced but perhaps causing different symptoms.

Treatment can take a long time – homoeopaths, for example, say that returning a patient completely to normal takes, on average, one month of treatment for every year that he has been ill. So it can be expensive. If there are several equally well-qualified acupuncturists near you, there is no harm in asking what they charge before you make an appointment. You may be surprised at the difference in prices. If you are enquiring about an ear stud, make sure that the acupuncturist will change it every two weeks, as this is essential to avoid infection.

Having made your appointment, what can you expect when you go for treatment? First of all, the acupuncturist will want to know about your present illness, your medical history, and your health in general. He will examine your tongue, pulse, skin and nails and will then make you comfortable on a couch or chair and insert the relevant needles.

As the needles go in, you may feel what is known as needling sensation, radiation or, in Chinese, deqi. It can take a number of forms – often a dull ache, but sometimes a tingling sensation. It should never be unpleasantly painful but can sometimes be quite fierce and may radiate a fairly long way. Sometimes patients feel slightly sick or light-headed at this point, but it only lasts a second or two. Some patients experience a warm glow travelling along the length of the meridian; occasionally this is accompanied by a flush on the skin. It is important to keep as still as possible while the needles are in to avoid dislodging them.

After the treatment, you may feel considerably better and often very relaxed. However, remember that you are not yet completely well. Sometimes a patient is so delighted at being relatively free of pain after a session of acupuncture that, despite warnings, she does more physical work than she should and sets herself back again. Having acupuncture treatment is like having a broken leg put into a cast. Once the plaster has set, the leg is comfortable and it may be possible, if you are careful, to walk with the aid of crutches. However, the leg is still broken inside its plaster cast and needs to be allowed to rest in order to heal properly. In the same way, if you have been ill for some time, the initial acupuncture treatments will not heal you right away – they will only start the energy flowing again. You need to be patient and work with the treatment, no matter how exciting the prospect might be of doing things that were previously impossible.

Occasionally, after a session of acupuncture, a patient's symptoms may become worse. This, surprisingly, is a good sign. It also occurs in other therapies, such as homoeopathy (where it is known as an aggravation) and in energy healing (where it is called a healing reaction). It is always a sign that the patient is going to respond well to treatment, so it should be an encouragement to continue, not an indication to give up. The reaction usually lasts twenty four hours or less and is often followed fairly quickly by a considerable improvement in the condition.

A session with an acupuncturist (or other complementary therapist) is longer and more relaxed that what we've come to expect from the average family doctor who is usually rushing to get through a waiting room full of patients. So take the opportunity to ask any questions you have about your treatment and about acupuncture in general.

While little use of acupuncture for anaesthesia is made in the West, it is possible to use it instead of pain-killers during childbirth. One great advantage, of course, is that it offers no risk to the baby. If you are pregnant and are interested in using acupuncture during labour, you need to speak to your midwife or obstetrician about it as well as your acupuncturist.

TRAINING TO BE AN ACUPUNCTURIST

If after reading about – and, perhaps, experiencing – acupuncture, you feel that you would like to train as an acupuncturist, there are now many courses available. When choosing a course, it is important to find one that is accredited so that you will be able to get registered once you have qualified. Nowadays, many of the courses available are affiliated to universities and offer degrees.

In the UK

In the UK there are seven fully accredited courses that meet the requirements of the British Acupuncture Accreditation Board (BAAB). They are:

The Acupuncture Academy
32 Hamilton Terrace, Leamington Spa CV32 4LY
01926 730284
https://www.theacupunctureacademy.org.uk/
Offering a Licentiate in Acupuncture (Lic.Ac.)

The City College of Acupuncture

55 East Rd, London N1 6AH

020 7253 1133

http://citycollegeofacupuncture.com/

Offering a Licentiate in Acupuncture (Lic.Ac.)

College of Integrated Chinese Medicine

19 Castle St, Reading RG1 7SB

0118 950 8880

https://www.acupuncturecollege.org.uk/

Offering a BSc (Hons) degree in acupuncture

International College of Oriental Medicine (ICOM)

Van Buren House, Green Hedges Avenue, East Grinstead RH19 1DZ

01342 313106

https://orientalmed.ac.uk/

Offering a Licentiate in Acupuncture (Lic.Ac.)

Northern College of Acupuncture

61 Micklegate, York YO1 6LJ

01904 343305

https://nca.ac.uk/

Offering a BSc (Hons) degree and an MSc degree in acupuncture

Lincoln College

Monks Rd, Lincoln LN2 5HQ

01522 876000

https://www.lincolncollege.ac.uk/

Offering a BSc (Hons) degree in acupuncture

University of Westminster
309 Regent St., London W1B 2HW
020 7911 5000
https://www.westminster.ac.uk/study
Offering a BSc (Hons) degree in acupuncture and Chinese medicine

In the USA and Canada

In North America there are around 50 acupuncture courses that are accredited by the Accreditation Commission for Acupuncture and Oriental Medicine (ACAOM) which, together with the Council of Colleges of Acupuncture and Oriental Medicine (CCAOM), was set up in 1982. These include:

Two in **Canada** (one in British Columbia, one in Ontario)
Three in **Arizona** (one in Phoenix, two in Tucson)
Fourteen in **California** (three in Los Angeles, the rest in Anaheim, Berkeley, Alhambra, Oakland, San Diego, San Francisco, Santa Cruz, San Jose, Santa Monica, Sunnyvale and Whittier)
Three in **Colorado** (Denver, Louisville and Boulder)
Six in **Florida** (two in Gainesville, the rest in Fort Lauderdale, Miami, Orlando and Sarasota)
Three in **Hawaii** (two in Honolulu, one in Kamuela)
Three in **Illinois** (two in Chicago, one in Lombard)
One in **Maryland** (Laurel)
One in **Massachusetts** (Newton)
Two in **Minnesota** (Bloomington and Roseville)
One in **New Jersey** (Bloomfield)
One in **New Mexico** (Santa Fe)
Eight in **New York** (five in New York City, the rest in Mineola, Seneca Falls and Syosset)

Two in **North Carolina** (Asheville and Sugar Grove)

Two in **Oregon** (both in Portland)

One in **Pennsylvania** (Glenside)

Three in **Texas** (two in Austin, one in Houston)

One in **Virginia** (Fairfax)

Two in **Washington** (Kenmore and Seattle)

One in **Wisconsin** (Racine)

For more details see https://www.acupuncturetoday.com/schools/

In Australia

In Australia, a number of courses are available. Five courses approved by the AACMA (Australian Acupuncture & Chinese Medicine Association) are:

Endeavour College of Natural Health
Campuses in NSW, Queensland, South Australia, Victoria & Western Australia
www.endeavour.edu.au/courses/bachelor-of-health-science-acupuncture
Offiering Bachelor of Health Science (Acupuncture)

RMIT University
Victoria
www.rmit.edu.au/programs
Offering Bachelor and Master degrees in Applied Science (Acupuncture)

Southern School of Natural Therapies
Campuses in Sydney, Melbourne, Brisbane, Adelaide, Southport and Leura
https://www.torrens.edu.au/about/our-heritage/ssnt
Offering Bachelor of Health Science (Chinese Medicine)

Sydney Institute of Traditional Chinese Medicine

www.sitcm.edu.au

Offering Bachelor of Traditional Chinese Medicine

Western Sydney University

www.westernsydney.edu.au/ssh

Offering Bachelor and Master degrees in Health Science

Made in United States
Cleveland, OH
06 November 2026

47647063R00101